THE ULTIMATE GUIDE TO PARENTING YOUR CHILD —— WITH —— AUTISM

AGES 4 TO 6

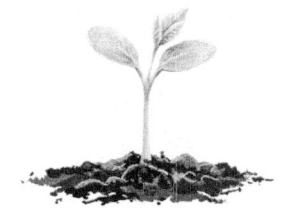

HEATHER KINGSLEY

© Copyright 2025—All rights reserved.

The content contained within this book may not be reproduced, duplicated or transmitted without direct written permission from the author or the publisher.

Under no circumstances will any blame or legal responsibility be held against the publisher, or author, for any damages, reparation, or monetary loss due to the information contained within this book, either directly or indirectly.

Legal Notice:

This book is copyright protected. It is only for personal use. You cannot amend, distribute, sell, use, quote or paraphrase any part, or the content within this book, without the consent of the author or publisher.

Disclaimer Notice:

Please note the information contained within this document is for educational and entertainment purposes only. All effort has been executed to present accurate, up to date, reliable, complete information. No warranties of any kind are declared or implied. Readers acknowledge that the author is not engaged in the rendering of legal, financial, medical or professional advice. The content within this book has been derived from various sources. Please consult a licensed professional before attempting any techniques outlined in this book.

By reading this document, the reader agrees that under no circumstances is the author responsible for any losses, direct or indirect, that are incurred as a result of the use of the information contained within this document, including, but not limited to, errors, omissions, or inaccuracies.

ALSO BY THE AUTHOR

THE ULTIMATE GUIDE TO PARENTING YOUR CHILD WITH AUTISM AGES 7-9
7 Key Steps to Support Your Child with ASD Build School Routines and Make Friends for Academic and Social Success

THE ULTIMATE GUIDE TO PARENTING YOUR CHILD WITH AUTISM AGES 10-12
9 Powerful Strategies to Help Your Child Gain Independence, Build Emotional Resilience, and Prepare for Puberty

THE ULTIMATE GUIDE TO PARENTING YOUR CHILD WITH AUTISM AGES 13-17
13 Advanced Strategies to Empower Your Teen with ASD to Overcome Social Challenges and Transition into Adulthood

THE ULTIMATE GUIDE TO PARENTING YOUR CHILD WITH AUTISM AGES 4-17 (4 BOOKS IN 1)
36 Proven Strategies to Help Your Child Thrive, Build Routines, Manage Meltdowns, and Achieve Long-Term Success

CONTENTS

Understanding the Icons 7

Introduction 9

1 | Understanding Autism in Early Childhood 13

2 | Building Effective Sensory Routines 25

3 | Emotional Regulation Made Simple 39

4 | Boosting Communication Skills Through Play 51

5 | Social Skills for Life 55

6 | School Readiness 77

7 | Promoting Independence and Confidence 91

8 | Managing Sensory Overload in Public Places 103

9 | Positive Reinforcement and Behavior Strategies 115

10| Long-Term Growth—Preparing for the Future 127

11 | Special Topics and Final Thoughts 139

Conclusion 149

Thank You! 153

Final Thank You 155

References 157

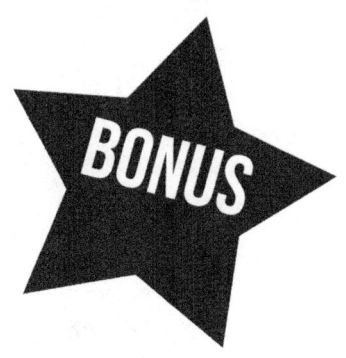

SPARK MP3 AUDIO AND QUICK START GUIDE

Unlock your child's potential!

Claim your free, personalized SPARK MP3 Audio and Quick Start Guide, designed specifically for your 4- to 6-year-old on the autism spectrum.

WHAT'S INCLUDED

This invaluable resource combines:

- **Age-appropriate affirmations** to build confidence, regulate emotions, and develop social skills.
- **Soothing classical music** by Mozart, Beethoven, Bach, and Pachelbel, to create a calming and supportive environment for your child.

HOW TO CLAIM YOUR FREE BONUS

1. **Visit:** https://www.ParentingMasterySeries.com/AutismBonus1/4-6, or

2. **Scan:** Scan the QR code below with your smartphone.

PERSONALIZE YOUR SPARK MP3

Once you're on the site you can tailor your SPARK MP3 to your child's unique needs by selecting a category of 20 affirmations:

- Focus areas **(SPARK)**:
  - **S**elf-Esteem & Confidence
  - **P**erseverance & Resilience
  - **A**cademics & Learning
  - **R**egulation & Emotion
  - **K**indness & Social Skills

Your child's SPARK MP3 Audio will arrive in your inbox within 3–5 days. You'll also get the Quick Start Guide, full of simple steps to help you use these affirmations at home.

Begin Your Child's Journey Today!

Empower your child to build confidence, achieve emotional balance, and thrive socially with this tailored resource designed to support you both.

Warmly, Heather

UNDERSTANDING THE ICONS

This guide uses 4 unique icons to highlight key information and make your reading experience easier. Here's what each one means:

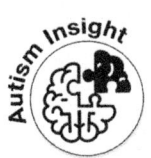
Autism Insight: Spotlight on autism-specific strategies and key insights. When you see this icon, you'll find advice and techniques tailored specifically to address challenges and opportunities for your child on the autism spectrum.

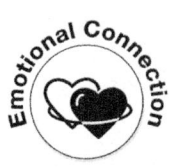
Emotional Connection: Stories and advice to foster empathy and understanding. This icon marks personal anecdotes, relatable scenarios, and emotional moments that provide deeper connections with autism.

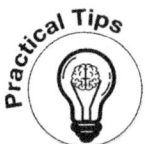
Practical Tips: Actionable advice and tools for immediate use. Look for this icon to discover clear, step-by-step recommendations or helpful tools you can apply immediately.

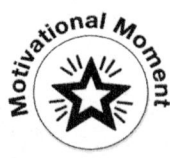 **Motivational Moment:** Inspiring and uplifting content to encourage you. This icon highlights moments meant to inspire you and remind you of every bit of progress and victory, no matter how small.

Tip: These icons are strategically placed throughout the book to help you navigate the most important content quickly and effectively.

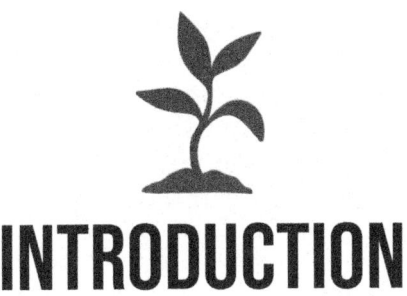

INTRODUCTION

Imagine standing at the edge of a vast, unpredictable landscape, unsure of which path to take. That's how parenting often feels—especially when your little one is navigating life on the autism spectrum. As a parent during these critical early years, you carry immense responsibility and encounter unique challenges. Yet, within the uncertainty shines a source of hope: your ability to turn everyday experiences into growth opportunities for your amazing little explorer.

Welcome to The Ultimate Guide to Parenting Your Child With Autism (Ages 4 to 6), where you'll find practical strategies, actionable solutions, and heartfelt support. This book exists to illuminate the road ahead, offering clear guidance through these transitional years. Early childhood is a pivotal time, full of developmental milestones that need nurturing support to help your 4- to 6-year-old flourish in meaningful ways. It's about unlocking their potential by building routines, enhancing social skills, and fostering emotional balance. This guide invites you to explore autism with clarity and compassion, finding ways to make everyday life enriching and fulfilling.

As a parent, you're already a hero in your little one's life. However, it's easy to feel overwhelmed by the overload of information out there or to feel underprepared for your child's unique abilities and needs. This guide offers a fresh approach—it cuts through the noise to provide actionable insights wrapped in empathy and understanding. Through a blend of personal anecdotes, current expert advice, proven strategies, and simplified concepts, you'll find practical ways to create consistency and foster a nurturing home and learning environment. The book focuses on age-specific needs, serving as a reliable roadmap for building meaningful connections.

Personal stories from parents who've walked this path can offer comfort and reassurance. They share both victories and setbacks, reminding you that you're not alone. As Kerry Magro, an award-winning national speaker on the spectrum, famously said, "Autism is not a tragedy. Ignorance is the tragedy." My hope is that this book equips you with not only knowledge but also confidence—a powerful tool to break down myths, set achievable expectations, and uncover often-overlooked possibilities.

This guide is carefully pieced together with thoughtful information at your fingertips, designed for even the busiest parents. It weaves together insights from current research and clinical practices, presenting them in a way that's easy to digest and apply. Each chapter concludes with key takeaways and simple exercises, giving you clear, actionable next steps.

You'll find strategies for creating sensory routines, building communication through play, managing transitions, and supporting positive behaviors while prioritizing your own well-being. The ultimate goal? To empower you with tools to expand your 4- to 6-year-old's world—and your own.

Parenting your son or daughter on the autism spectrum takes resilience, understanding, patience, and love. This book balances practical solutions with emotional inspiration, offering more than just guidance—it's meant to be your sidekick on this whimsical adventure. Some moments will test your resolve, while others will bring joy, warmth, and immense pride.

Self-care is key. Taking care of yourself replenishes your energy while shifting you to the right headspace so you can take on anything, big or small. Together, we'll explore techniques to kick guilt to the curb, fight through exhaustion, and experience burnout less often through mindfulness and self-compassion. Picture a moment when your mindful intervention helps your child flourish like never before. Imagine guiding them through challenges, celebrating breakthroughs, and viewing every victory as a step forward for both of you. This isn't just a vision—it's achievable with structured guidance tailored to your 4- to 6-year-old.

My seven-step framework breaks the process into manageable segments, ensuring you have a reliable method without feeling overwhelmed.

By picking up this book, you've already taken a huge step toward empowering yourself and your family. Each page brings you closer to understanding your child and fully embracing their identity with assurance and strength. Let's create a reality where autism becomes one small facet of their uniqueness, not an impossible challenge. With practical strategies for managing sensory challenges and building routines, this book helps you unlock their full potential.

Are you ready to elevate both of your lives and go from surviving to thriving? Get ready to turn the page with courage, hope, and determination in your back pocket. Together, we'll foster an environment where they not only prosper but also shine—because nothing's more rewarding than seeing your kiddo reach for the stars they're destined for.

Each step you take strengthens your ability to create an environment where they can truly shine.

UNDERSTANDING AUTISM IN EARLY CHILDHOOD

WHAT YOU NEED TO KNOW ABOUT YOUR 4 TO 6 YEAR-OLD

Understanding autism in early childhood involves observing unique behaviors that may emerge as your 4- to 6-year-old grows and develops. As a parent, whether you're just starting this journey or already have experience but still face challenges, you may often find yourself moving through a maze of unfamiliar communication styles and behaviors exhibited by your child. Recognizing these patterns is important for fostering better understanding and offering the supportive environment they need. Whether you're picking up on nonverbal cues, understanding emotional responses, or identifying preferences for solitary play, your awareness as a parent plays a pivotal role in developing effective communication with them. The process thrives on patience and observation, encouraging you to embrace their unique expressions and reinforce them in ways that cater to their comfort and growth.

As you look deeper into this chapter, you'll explore various strategies aimed at recognizing specific behavioral patterns exhibited by your child in this age group. From understanding how nonverbal communication manifests to deciphering emotional responses, each section provides insights into how autism can appear during early childhood. You'll uncover how communication aids can bridge gaps, discover the value of parallel play for gentle social integration, and see how consistent daily routines support your 4- to 6-year-old's development. This chapter provides you with practical intervention strategies tailored to their needs. By applying these strategies, you can transform your understanding into actionable steps, building a foundation for meaningful connections and smoother transitions.

RECOGNIZING BEHAVIORAL PATTERNS SPECIFIC TO AGES 4 TO 6

In maneuvering the early years of parenting your child on the autism spectrum, you'll often face challenges in understanding their unique communication styles and behaviors. One of the key elements to focus on is nonverbal communication. Children on the autism spectrum often use nonverbal cues to express themselves. This may include gestures, facial expressions, or even body movements that convey their thoughts and emotions. Noticing these subtle signals is key to understanding their needs. By doing so, you can better understand what they're trying to communicate and respond in a way that makes them feel heard and understood. Incorporating visual communication aids, such as pictures or sign language, helps bridge communication gaps and creates meaningful connections.

Another common characteristic is a preference for solitary play over group activities. While this tendency may seem concerning, it reflects your 4- to 6-year-old's unique social needs. Group interactions can sometimes be overwhelming, and the need for space often indicates that your child is seeking comfort in familiar surroundings. You can gently support them by introducing opportunities for parallel play, where they engage alongside peers without direct interaction. This approach eases them into more socially engaging environments over time. Respecting their need for space helps create a safe and supportive setting for gradual social growth.

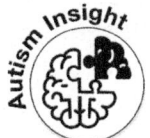

Emotional responses in your child with autism can greatly differ from those of their neurotypical peers. Some might exhibit intense emotional reactions to everyday situations, while others might show quieter responses. It's crucial for you, as the parent, to recognize these distinct patterns and develop tailored strategies to provide emotional support. Understanding that their emotional response is part of their communication opens up pathways for effective parenting. For example, if they're distressed during transitions, providing clear verbal cues ahead of time or using a visual schedule can help manage expectations and reduce anxiety. Regularly discussing emotions and validating your son or daughter's feelings nurtures a supportive environment where they feel safe to express themselves.

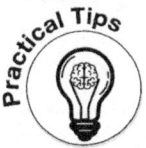

Consistency in daily routines offers another layer of predictability that your 4- to 6-year-old may find comforting. A well-structured environment caters to their preference for routine and helps reduce stress. Children who thrive on predictable schedules often feel more relaxed when they know what to expect throughout the day. This predictability might include maintaining consistent mealtimes, bedtime rituals, or lining up a specific sequence of activities before transitioning to a new task. Visual planners or charts, using symbols or pictures to represent activities, give your child a sense of control and anticipation over their daily experiences.

While recognizing these behaviors can initially seem like a lot of work, it's important to remember that these patterns are unique expressions of your young adventurer's individual personality and needs. Recording their behavior, including triggers for distress or joy, provides valuable insights over time. Sharing these observations with healthcare professionals can aid in crafting personalized intervention plans tailored to support their developmental trajectory. Engaging with trusted pediatricians or therapists can offer additional guidance, helping you adopt strategies that align with your child's individual strengths and struggles.

Ultimately, the journey involves an ongoing process of learning and adaptation. Each step gives you deeper insight into your kid's world. Resources like support groups, educational workshops, and counseling services can be instrumental in building a network of understanding and reassurance for families. Embracing a community that shares experiences and advice can alleviate feelings of isolation and foster a collaborative approach to overcoming challenges.

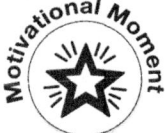 Your love and resilience as a parent play a critical role in shaping your child's growth and development. When you focus on small, manageable goals, you and your family can celebrate progress, no matter how minor it may seem. These achievements build a strong foundation for fostering self-confidence and independence in your young learner on the autism spectrum, empowering them to navigate the world with greater assurance.

TAILORING INTERVENTIONS FOR YOUR CHILD AGED 4 TO 6

When addressing autism in early childhood, it's important to understand that a personalized approach based on your child's unique strengths and challenges is vital. Every kid on the autism spectrum is different, which means that effective strategies need to be tailored specifically to them. What works for one child may not be suitable for another, highlighting the importance of recognizing these differences to ensure interventions are meaningful and relevant.

Personalized strategies start with identifying what makes your kiddo exceptional. Focus on their strengths—perhaps in memory, creativity, or problem-solving—and recognize their challenges, like communication difficulties or sensory sensitivities. For example, if your 4- to 6-year-old excels in visual learning, they might benefit from picture-based communication tools, while another child with strong auditory skills may thrive with song or verbal interactions. These insights will guide you in developing strategies that leverage their strengths while addressing areas that need support.

Creating customized goals is another critical aspect of personalizing interventions for your child. Goals should be realistic and aligned with their individual abilities, helping to foster motivation instead of frustration. When you set attainable milestones, it makes progress more visible and reinforces positive outcomes. For instance, if they enjoy drawing but struggle with social interaction, a goal could focus on using art to strengthen communication with peers. This approach builds on existing skills and encourages growth in other areas through activities that capture their interest.

As you guide their development, remember that their needs and capabilities will change over time, so it's important to be flexible with your strategies. A strategy that works at age 4 may need adjustment by the time they turn 6, as new skills emerge and challenges evolve. This dynamic process requires you to continually assess and adapt your approach, making sure that your interventions remain relevant and supportive. Regular evaluations help you recalibrate objectives, introduce new techniques, or phase out methods that no longer serve your child's best interests. This adaptability helps maintain momentum in their development and prevents stagnation.

Your family dynamics are essential in supporting these tailored interventions. Engaging everyone in the therapeutic process can strengthen overall development. Family members provide invaluable insights into your child's behaviors, preferences, and responses, offering a comprehensive view that informs your intervention strategies. When you and other family members actively participate, it creates a supportive environment where interventions are reinforced outside of formal sessions.

For instance, practicing communication exercises at home extends the benefits of therapy into everyday life, making progress more sustainable.

Even involving siblings in playful activities can promote inclusion and understanding, nurturing an environment of acceptance and support within your family. Seeking resources like workshops, support groups, or consultations equips everyone with the tools needed to contribute confidently. This empowerment not only aids your son or daughter's development but also strengthens family bonds, creating a nurturing space where everyone plays a role in their progress.

Incorporating a personalized approach means considering both present circumstances and future needs. As your child grows and learns, their world expands, introducing new challenges and opportunities. You always have to be one step ahead of the game, which seems a bit daunting, but that's ok! You'll figure out how to tackle this part of the process in no time. There will be a time when they approach school age—preparing them for social settings and structured environments ahead of time is one way to make sure you're preparing them for the future instead of throwing them in the deep end. Personalized strategies might include practice scenarios at home or joining small-group interactions to ease this transition smoothly.

THE BENEFITS OF STARTING EARLY

Engaging in early intervention for autism can significantly enhance your child's developmental outcomes. Timely support and practices offer both immediate and long-term benefits. Research shows that starting intervention strategies during early childhood, especially between the ages of 4 and 6, helps children improve communication and socialization skills, enhances cognitive abilities, and adopts more adaptive behaviors (Daniolou et al., 2022). These improvements greatly contribute to their overall well-being and sense of independence as they grow.

One major benefit of starting early intervention is that it helps establish foundational skills. At this developmental stage, your 4- to 6-year-old is particularly open to learning new skills in a structured and supportive environment. Focusing on key areas like language and communication helps lay essential building blocks that support future transitions. Activities designed to improve joint attention and imitation skills are great examples because both are crucial for social interactions and learning. Building these foundational skills early can support their immediate growth and prepare them for challenges they may face as they get older.

To maximize the benefits of early interventions, you should actively engage in supportive practices. When you participate in these programs, you'll become more confident and knowledgeable about your child's needs and how to address them. Your involvement helps them apply what they've learned at home or in therapy to new situations. This engagement not only boosts their progress but also helps you feel reassured and proactive in your parenting journey.

Another key aspect of early intervention is facilitating your access to resources and support networks as soon as possible. Taking advantage of these resources early on can be transformative for you and your family as you handle the complexities of raising a child on the autism spectrum. Support networks provide invaluable emotional support and practical advice, connecting you with professionals who specialize in autism care. Exploring community programs, online resources, and local services tailored to autism can help you find guidance that aligns with your kid's needs. These connections can also lead to discovering funding opportunities for specialized therapies or educational programs, helping to alleviate some financial pressures.

When implementing early intervention strategies, it's important to recognize the diversity in the effectiveness of various methods. While results may vary based on individual needs and circumstances, research consistently highlights the potential for developmental advancements through targeted early intensive behavioral interventions (Franz et al., 2022). These interventions, often recommended for around 25 to 40 hours per week, involve a mix of play-based and structured activities aimed at nurturing critical skills in your 4- to 6-year-old. These programs are known to be effective in fostering improvements in multiple domains, enhancing their capacity to thrive in everyday environments.

Establishing a routine that incorporates consistent intervention and learning opportunities creates an environment where they can thrive. This routine could include regular sessions with therapists, structured play at home, or participation in group activities designed to promote social interaction. Routine offers predictability, which your child may find comforting, making them more receptive to new experiences and challenges. Through consistency and repetition, skills learned during formal interventions can become part of their daily habits and actions.

As you start down this path, it's worth considering the role technology can play in supporting your early intervention efforts. Tools such as communication apps, educational games, and behavior-tracking software can be seamlessly integrated into your day-to-day routines. These tools not only aid in strengthening skills learned during therapy sessions but also provide you with a way to monitor progress and make adjustments as needed. Technology can serve as a bridge between you and your loved one by offering innovative communication tools and interactive learning opportunities, making the intervention process even more enriching.

The path of early intervention is multifaceted and requires careful consideration of your child's unique needs and abilities. Collaborating closely with teams of healthcare providers, educators, and therapists who share a common goal of supporting their development is very important. Regular assessments and ongoing adjustments to intervention plans ensure that practices remain relevant and effective over time. By embracing a collaborative approach, you'll build a robust support system that maximizes developmental opportunities.

FINAL INSIGHTS

Understanding how autism appears in your child offers helpful insights for navigating this journey effectively. In this chapter, we talked about the unique ways kids on the autism spectrum express themselves, often through nonverbal communication like gestures and facial expressions. By keeping a close eye on these cues, you can better understand their needs and support them effectively. Strategies for encouraging social interaction, such as parallel play, help your 4- to 6-year-old gradually adapt to group settings. Tailoring interventions to suit their individual strengths, whether through visual aids or small milestones, empowers your child to grow at their own pace. The importance of collaboration between families and professionals ensure that interventions remain relevant and supportive throughout their overall development.

When you approach early intervention with a personalized

mindset, you enrich the developmental outcome for your child. Starting early can make a big difference, fostering the foundations for relevant skills and providing you with the confidence needed to support their progress. Recognizing different emotional responses and establishing consistent routines play crucial roles in nurturing a sense of security and growth. Accessing support networks and resources allows you to provide comprehensive care while integrating technology introduces new avenues for learning and communication. Overall, creating a nurturing environment that adapts to their evolving needs encourages both immediate growth and long-term success, helping your family feel more supported on this path.

Next, we'll focus on the importance of building sensory routines to help your 4- to 6-year-old manage and regulate their emotions and environment.

KEY TAKEAWAYS

- **Recognizing nonverbal communication:** Observe gestures, facial expressions, and body language to better understand your 4- to 6-year-old's needs.
- **The importance of routine and consistency:** Use visual schedules and consistent routines to reduce stress and create a sense of security.
- **Encourage parallel play:** Introduce social settings gradually by having your child play alongside others without direct interaction.
- **Tailoring interventions:** Personalize strategies to suit their strengths, using visual aids or small milestones to support progress.
- **Start early intervention:** Focus on developing communication, social, and adaptive skills between ages 4 and 6 for long-term growth.

BUILDING EFFECTIVE SENSORY ROUTINES

Building effective sensory routines is essential for you and your 4- to 6-year-old, especially as they navigate the challenges of emotional regulation. Sensory experiences play a crucial role in shaping how they connect with their environment and build confidence in daily interactions. As a parent, you might feel like you're always learning and adapting, working to understand your child's unique needs and creating a space where they feel supported. Understanding the pillars of an effective sensory routine can support emotional regulation while creating a nurturing environment where your 4- to 6-year-old feels understood and secure.

By focusing on the key elements of an effective sensory routine, you'll help your little one on the autism spectrum regulate their emotions and build a sense of safety and understanding of their surroundings. In this chapter, you'll discover how personalized sensory routines can support individual needs. We'll explore how to recognize sensory-seeking and sensory-avoiding behaviors and provide strategies tailored to their preferences. These insights aim to empower you with the tools to create environments where they can flourish both emotionally and developmentally.

IDENTIFYING SENSORY-SEEKING VS. SENSORY-AVOIDING BEHAVIORS

Understanding the different ways your young learner processes sensory input can feel challenging, especially when it comes to recognizing sensory-seeking and sensory-avoiding behaviors. However, recognizing these behaviors is key to crafting effective sensory routines that help build emotional balance and resilience.

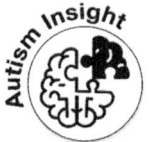
Start by figuring out their unique sensory profile. Sensory-seeking behaviors might include constant movement, touching everything, or seeking loud noises, whereas sensory-avoiding behaviors may involve covering their ears at loud sounds, avoiding certain textures, or being startled by bright lights. Your child might exhibit traits from both categories depending on their circumstances or state of mind.

Differentiating between whether they are sensory-seeking or sensory-avoiding is key to developing tailored interventions that match your little explorer's needs. For example, if they seek sensory input, activities like jumping on a trampoline or playing with textured toys can provide the stimulation they need. On the other hand, if they tend to avoid sensory experiences, your young learner might benefit from a calm, clutter-free space, and soothing activities designed to minimize overwhelming stimuli. These personalized strategies help make daily experiences more manageable and support emotional well-being.

Maintaining a sensory journal can be a great method for creating interventions that are personalized for your son or daughter—helping you track your child's reactions to various sensory inputs, identifying triggers, and developing coping strategies. This systematic approach enables better decision-making in adapting to environments at home or school. Consulting professionals, like an occupational therapist, can further assess their sensory processing and recommend targeted interventions. Collaborating with experts strengthens your support network, ensuring you receive the most suitable care and guidance for their needs.

Understanding your little one's sensory preferences isn't just about addressing immediate needs; it's about proactively planning for everyday activities and establishing long-term strategies to improve both their and your family's quality of life. Knowing which types of sensory input they prefer or find challenging can help shape decisions about your home's layout and activity choices. For example, this knowledge can help guide choices in their clothing, food, and even social activities, creating an environment where they feel cozy and safe.

Recognizing signs of sensory overload is another important aspect. Overload occurs when your child's brain is bombarded with too much sensory information at once, potentially leading to stress, anxiety, or meltdowns. Symptoms may include restlessness, physical discomfort, or an urgent need to escape the sensory source or situation (Pfeiffer et al., 2011). Identifying these signs early is crucial. You might need to remove them from the overstimulating environment, provide a quiet place for them to regroup, or offer calming items from a sensory toolkit.

Sensory Tool Kits

A sensory tool kit for your 4- to 6-year-old can be incredibly helpful in supporting their sensory needs and emotional regulation. Here's a breakdown of what to include, tailored to various sensory preferences and modalities:

- **Tactile Tools:**
  - Fidget toys: Soft stress balls, textured fidgets, or squishy toys can help with self-soothing.

- Playdough or putty: These engage your child in calming, repetitive motions and help build fine motor skills.
- Weighted items: A small, weighted blanket or lap pad can provide deep pressure, helping them feel grounded.
- Soft fabrics: A small piece of soft, comforting fabric to hold or rub can be very soothing.

- **Auditory Tools:**
  - Noise-canceling headphones: These are useful for reducing overwhelming background noise.
  - Calming music or sounds: A playlist of gentle tunes or nature sounds can provide an auditory escape.
  - Sound machines: Devices that offer white noise, ocean waves, or other calming sounds can assist during transitions or bedtime.

- **Visual Tools:**
  - Liquid motion toys: These slow-moving, visually captivating toys can help your child focus and relieve stress.
  - Light-up toys: Visual stimulation like soft, glowing toys or a small LED projector can engage them without overwhelming their senses.
  - Picture schedules: Visuals help them understand routines, reducing anxiety during transitions.

- **Body Awareness Tools:**
  - Body socks: These stretchy, enclosed fabric suits provide resistance, helping your child feel their bodily movements.
  - Therapy ball: Sitting or bouncing gently on a ball can offer sensory input and movement.
  - Crash pads or bean bags: Perfect for rough-and-tumble play, these provide a safe space to jump and crash.

- **Oral Tools:**
  - Chewable necklaces: Safe, non-toxic silicone necklaces or bracelets can meet their need to chew.

- Flavorful snacks: Having a variety of crunchy, chewy, or cold snacks like pretzels, gummies, or cold fruit provides effective oral stimulation.

- **Movement Tools:**
  - Swing or hammock: If possible, having a swing or hammock available provides soothing and rhythmic movement.
  - Balance board: Encourages gentle rocking or balancing for sensory stimulation.
  - Jump rope or small trampoline: Great for high-energy young learners who need to burn off extra energy in a controlled way.

This tool kit can be easily adapted to fit their specific needs, and it's great to have portable options for outings or school.

Proactively preparing for situations that could cause sensory overload is essential. For example, planning outings during quieter times, ensuring they get enough rest beforehand, and having an exit strategy can make outings more enjoyable for everyone involved. Sharing information with others, such as teachers or family members, about their sensory needs helps ensure consistent support in various settings.

INCORPORATING CALMING ACTIVITIES INTO DAILY ROUTINES

Integrating calming activities into your daily routine is one of the best ways to help manage their emotions, particularly between the ages of 4 and 6. This strategy is especially beneficial for children on the autism spectrum because it offers a stable environment that reduces anxiety and enhances emotional well-being. You can adopt various calming strategies, each tailored to fit individual sensory preferences.

One effective approach is to formulate a personalized sensory routine to alleviate anxiety. By observing their reactions to different stimuli, you can incorporate soothing elements into their daily schedule. For example, they may find comfort in soft textures, like a plush toy or blanket, and could also respond positively to calming sounds, such as soothing music or white noise. When you identify these preferences, you're able to create an environment that supports their emotional needs. Engaging in quiet time activities, such as reading together or working on a simple puzzle, can also help promote relaxation.

Real Life Story: Martinez Family

The Martinez family had been managing challenges ever since their five-year-old daughter, Lily, was diagnosed with autism. Everyday events like certain textures, loud noises, or bright lights often led to meltdowns, leaving them feeling lost and unsure of how to help. After a particularly rough day, Lily's mother, Julia, began keeping a sensory journal, tracking everything from Lily's activities to the triggers that caused her stress. Slowly, patterns emerged—bright lights or crowded spaces heightened Lily's anxiety, while soft blankets, calming music, and chewable toys brought her comfort.

With this new understanding, the family transformed their home into a sensory-friendly space, complete with noise-canceling headphones, weighted blankets, and fidget toys. They also worked with Lily's teacher to create a sensory corner at school for her breaks. The change was transformative—Lily's meltdowns became less frequent and shorter, and she found more joy in her daily life. Even car rides, which had been a major challenge, were now manageable with her sensory kit filled with her favorite calming tools. The sensory journal provided the family with valuable insights, enabling them to support Lily in ways that made a meaningful difference.

Julia's decision to keep a sensory journal allowed the family to discover Lily's sensory preferences and patterns, helping them make adjustments that better suited her needs.

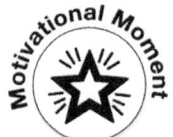

Scheduling calming strategies throughout the day can help reduce stress during transitions, like moving from playtime to dinner, by adding a sense of predictability and security. Incorporating familiar routines and using a visual schedule helps your 4- to 6-year-old better anticipate upcoming activities, making transitions smoother. Mindfulness practices, such as deep breathing or guided imagery, can also build emotional awareness and provide additional support. For instance, practicing mindfulness together strengthens your bond, creating a safe and supportive space for them to express feelings. In challenging moments, holding their hand and taking deep breaths together can bring comfort and calm to both of you.

Evaluating the long-term effectiveness of calming activities is imperative, and keeping a sensory journal can track your child's responses and highlight strategies that work best for them. This ongoing practice enables you to monitor changes, refine routines, and ensure that interventions remain effective as they grow. Regular evaluation tailors activities to meet their changing needs. Regularly consulting professionals, such as an occupational therapist or a pediatric psychologist, can offer valuable assessments and guidance, enhancing sensory routines and introducing tailored strategies to support your young learner's development effectively.

USING EVERYDAY OBJECTS AS SENSORY TOOLS

When it comes to building effective sensory routines for your curious explorer, using everyday items already in your home can be both practical and innovative. The idea is to create an engaging environment that fosters their emotional regulation without the need for expensive or specialized tools.

Household items like dried rice, beans, pasta, or even simple objects like sponges, old magazines, or cardboard boxes can serve as excellent resources for sensory play. For instance, a simple bowl of dried rice can become a treasure hunt where your kiddo can find toys hidden within, engaging their senses while developing fine motor skills. As they dig, pour, and sift through these materials, they're exploring new textures while learning to manipulate objects with precision. This tactile interaction strengthens their hand-eye coordination and dexterity, which are essential skills for daily activities like dressing themselves or handling utensils.

Sensory play using these common items naturally builds curiosity and comfort. Offering a variety of textures and forms to interact with creates opportunities for exploration within a familiar setting. Your child might enjoy crumpling magazine pages, which produce different sounds and textures. These interactions serve as an invitation for them to uncover their world more deeply, promoting cognitive growth as they connect cause and effect through experimentation and observation.

Beyond the physical aspects, interactions with ordinary objects can bolster their independence and confidence. For example, demonstrating how to use a sponge to draw patterns in water can inspire them to recreate the activity on their own. Such activities build a sense of accomplishment, boosting their confidence and reinforcing their ability to learn and adapt.

While creativity and resourcefulness are key in crafting these opportunities, safety must remain a priority. Avoid sharp objects, small parts that could be swallowed, or any materials that might cause allergic reactions. Always supervise playtime to ensure that your child uses the items safely, and maintain a clean and organized play area to prevent accidents.

Providing a safe exploratory environment is imperative not just for physical safety but also for emotional security. A controlled environment, where outcomes are predictable and guidance is consistent, helps your child feel at ease. This trust creates the groundwork for a secure attachment, which is fundamental to healthy emotional development.

BUILDING EFFECTIVE SENSORY ROUTINES

By integrating sensory play with regular household items into daily routines, you can effectively support their emotional regulation. These activities don't require extensive planning or special tools; instead, they rely on simple creativity and awareness of their individual sensory needs. Rather than striving for a "perfect" sensory tool, consider that nearly anything can serve this purpose if viewed through a sensory-friendly lens.

Additionally, the simplicity of these items encourages spontaneous play, which often leads to them being more engaged. Without the need for a strict agenda or structure, activities can flow naturally based on their unique interests and responses. This organic form of play allows them to progress at their own pace, making learning enjoyable rather than a task.

Including siblings or peers can only make this experience more grand. Group play scenarios, such as creating a "feely box" from an old shoe box filled with textured objects like feathers, cotton balls, and gravel, promote social skills. During these interactions, your little one will practice sharing, turn-taking, and communicating their discoveries, creating a collaborative spirit within them. Activities that utilize simple, shared materials build a communal atmosphere where your little one and others learn valuable lessons about teamwork and empathy.

While engaging your 4- to 6-year-old in sensory play using household items may seem straightforward, the positive impact can be profound. These activities provide a foundation for physical, cognitive, and emotional growth, supporting overall development. Furthermore, they offer a reassuring framework for you, as a parent, to nurture their abilities within the comfort of your own home. Allowing them to engage with their environment in a manner that suits their developmental stage and individual preferences is fundamental to building a resilient, self-assured learner who approaches challenges with enthusiasm and confidence.

FINAL INSIGHTS

In this chapter, we explored the importance of understanding sensory-seeking and sensory-avoiding behaviors in your 4- to 6-year-old. Identifying these behaviors allows you to create personalized sensory routines that help them regulate their emotions.

Creating a supportive environment is key to fostering healthy development. Encourage sensory exploration through familiar objects, allowing for mindful play that suits their unique needs. By prioritizing these sensory routines, you foster emotional growth and overall well-being while creating a home environment where they feel secure and supported.

Now it's time to move on to the next chapter, where we'll chat about emotional regulation.

KEY TAKEAWAYS

- **Understand sensory profiles:** Recognizing whether your 4- to 6-year-old seeks or avoids sensory input helps you tailor routines.
- **Maintain a sensory journal:** Track their reactions to identify triggers and effective calming strategies.
- **Utilize sensory tool kits:** Include tactile, auditory, and visual tools to address their needs.
- **Incorporate everyday objects:** Use household items for sensory play, encouraging curiosity and confidence.
- **Create calming routines:** Predictable schedules and mindfulness help reduce stress and anxiety.

REVISIT YOUR FREE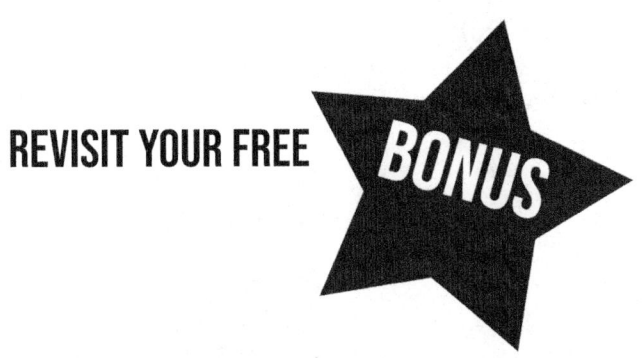

SPARK MP3 AUDIO AND QUICK START GUIDE

As you've learned in this chapter, emotional regulation is a vital skill for your child on the autism spectrum. To help you put these strategies into action, I've created the **SPARK MP3 Audio and Quick Start Guide**, a free, personalized resource designed specifically for your child aged 4 to 6.

WHY SPARK MP3 CAN HELP YOUR CHILD

- **Boosts Confidence:** Inspires self-belief with positive age-appropriate affirmations.
- **Promotes Emotional Balance:** Helps them manage emotions and reduces sensory overload.
- **Builds Social Skills:** Encourages kindness and empathy in a calming, enjoyable way.

The SPARK MP3 features 20 affirmations paired with soothing classical music, creating a supportive experience tailored to your child's needs. The Quick Start Guide provides simple, actionable steps to integrate it seamlessly into your daily routine.

CLAIM YOUR FREE BONUS NOW

If you haven't already, take a moment to claim your free SPARK MP3 Audio:

1. **Visit:** https://www.ParentingMasterySeries.com/Autism Bonus1/4-6, or

2. **Scan:** Scan the QR code below with your smart phone

PERSONALIZE YOUR SPARK MP3

Once you're on the site you can tailor your SPARK MP3 to your child's unique needs by selecting a category of 20 affirmations:

- Focus areas (**SPARK**):
    - **S**elf-Esteem & Confidence
    - **P**erseverance & Resilience
    - **A**cademics & Learning
    - **R**egulation & Emotion
    - **K**indness & Social Skills

Your personalized SPARK MP3 Audio will land directly in your inbox in **3–5 days** along with the **Quick Start Guide** to help you get started.

Help Your Child Thrive Today!

Empower your child with this powerful tool designed to boost their confidence, balance emotions, and build social skills—all in a fun, calming way!

Warmly, Heather

3
EMOTIONAL REGULATION MADE SIMPLE

Emotional regulation is a skill that, once mastered, can transform the way you interact with your 4- to 6-year-old. By breaking it into manageable steps, you'll help them better manage their emotions and create an environment where both of you can grow and succeed, despite daily challenges. Recognizing early signs of emotional upheaval and understanding the unique triggers of your young learner on the autism spectrum can ease the stress you carry.

As we move to this next chapter, you'll discover a bundle of emotional regulation techniques designed specifically for these challenges. These methods aren't just theoretical; they're practical tools that you can use in everyday scenarios to help your little one effectively regulate their emotions.

Recognizing Early Signs of Emotional Dysregulation

Parenting a 4- to 6-year-old on the autism spectrum can feel overwhelming at times. I'm here to tell you that you're doing an incredible job, even on days when it feels hard to keep up. Recognizing emotional dysregulation can make a huge difference, offering you a sense of clarity when venturing into uncharted territory. Now seems like a good time to go over some of the early signs of emotional dysregulation together.

PHYSICAL CUES

Your young learner might not be able to tell you how they're feeling with words, but their body can tell you so much. Watch for subtle physical changes, like fidgeting more than usual, withdrawing into themselves, or clenching their fists and stiffening their posture. These are signs that their emotional distress is building up. Think of it as watching the sky darken before a storm. The key here is heightened awareness—catching these cues early gives you the upper hand, allowing you to step in with soothing strategies before their emotions spiral.

EMOTIONAL VOCABULARY

You might be amazed at how much it helps when your 4- to 6-year-old has the words to express what's going on inside. Begin with simple words like "mad," "sad," or "scared" to give them a way to communicate what they're feeling before they're overwhelmed. A feelings chart or emotion flashcards can be lifesavers here. The more they learn to name their emotions, the less they'll need to scream or shut down. Think of it as giving them the tools to navigate their own emotional landscape, and over time, those little victories will add up.

ROUTINE CHANGES

Routine is your best friend, but any shift in that routine can send a young learner's anxiety through the roof. For example, small changes, such as going to a new store or skipping their usual snack time, may cause distress. The more you recognize how these changes affect their emotional state, the better prepared you'll be. If you know a transition is coming, give them a heads-up. Visual schedules or timers can help them anticipate what's next. It's all about managing their expectations and offering consistency, which helps them feel safe and secure.

Real Life Story: Tom and Mathew

Tom had always prided himself on being a hands-on dad, but when his son Mathew, aged 4, was diagnosed with autism, Tom found himself overwhelmed by the emotional meltdowns that seemed to erupt out of nowhere. Mathew's frustration was heartbreaking. He would bang his fists on the floor, scream, or become physically restless, unable to explain what he needed. It was exhausting, and Tom often felt powerless.

One day, after an especially rough afternoon, Tom confided in Mathew's therapist, who suggested watching Mathew's subtle physical cues—small signs that came before the outbursts. The therapist assured him that progress was possible, even if it felt like nothing was changing.

Tom began to notice subtle signs, such as when Mathew would clench his fists, fidget excessively, or refuse to sit still. Calmly, Tom would bring out a soothing blanket Mathew loved and offer him two simple words: "sad" and "eat." Mathew often became upset if he was hungry. Slowly but surely, Mathew began to connect these words with his feelings. When Mathew was on the verge of frustration, Tom would show him the cue cards, and Mathew learned to identify his needs. "Sad," Mathew would say when he felt overwhelmed, or "Eat," when hunger made him upset. It wasn't overnight, but day by day, they were building a bridge of understanding, and for the first time, Tom felt like he was truly helping Mathew navigate the big feelings inside.

PREVENTATIVE AND RESPONSIVE STRATEGIES

The balance between preventing and responding is key. When you recognize these early signs—whether it's a known trigger, a physical cue, or an unexpected routine change—you're already ahead of the game. By stepping in early, you can often de-escalate situations before they intensify. Even when a meltdown happens, you'll feel more prepared to respond calmly, using soothing strategies such as deep breathing, sensory tools, or positive reinforcement.

Developing patience and empathy for your child's emotional dysregulation is crucial, as their episodes often stem from difficulty processing emotions rather than misbehavior. Responding with compassion and validating their feelings can help model emotionally intelligent behavior and show them that their emotions are understood. As they grow, they'll begin to mirror this behavior, developing strong emotional intelligence.

Finally, consistently reinforcing positive behavior is vital. While addressing emotional dysregulation, celebrate when your child successfully communicates feelings or copes with change. This could be as simple as offering verbal praise or a sticker as a reward for efforts made toward self-regulation. Acknowledging these small successes builds confidence and encourages further growth.

Teaching Calming Strategies for Self-Regulation

Did you know that simple breathing exercises can be a powerful tool for you and your 4- to 6-year-old on the autism spectrum to manage emotions effectively together? Introducing these techniques as fun and interactive activities encourages your son or daughter to pause and take deep breaths, taking their anxiety during emotional moments down a few notches. For instance, try an exercise like "blowing out birthday candles," where they pretend their fingers are candles and blow each one out slowly, helping them focus on measured, calming breaths.

Another playful technique is "balloon breaths," where you both pretend to inflate a balloon by cupping your hands in front of your mouths and gradually expanding them with every inhale, then deflating the balloon on the exhale. These simple activities turn breathing exercises into engaging games, teaching them the benefits of controlled breathing in a way that feels natural and enjoyable.

Mindfulness practices are another critical component of helping your young learner handle emotions. Encouraging present-moment awareness allows them to become more aware of their feelings, helping them to recognize and accept emotions rather than feeling completely defeated. Simple exercises, like imagining their favorite color or visualizing a calming place, help with concentration and focus. A useful example is the "5-4-3-2-1 senses" exercise, where they identify:

- 5 things they can see
- 4 things they can hear
- 3 things they can smell
- 2 things they can touch
- 1 thing they can taste

This grounding activity creates a buffer between a stimulus and a reaction, reducing impulsivity during emotional flare-ups.

Establishing predictable calming routines as a family can reinforce security and nurture self-regulation. Routines, like nightly wind-downs that include reading, listening to short stories, or meditation, create comforting boundaries, reducing uncertainties that may trigger emotional distress. Including the entire family in these routines fosters stronger bonds and emotional well-being for everyone.

Encourage independence by inviting your child to choose how they participate, fostering their sense of ownership and personal growth. After emotional experiences, having follow-up discussions can help them reflect and build emotional intelligence.

When introducing these strategies, start with techniques that resonate most with your child's interests and age. Gradually incorporate new practices as they become comfortable with the initial ones to expand their emotional regulation tools. Visual aids, such as images of breathing exercises or calming scenes, can further enhance the experience—especially for visual learners.

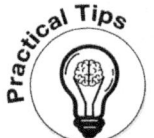

Creating a Calming Toolbox

Think of the calming toolbox as a personalized kit filled with resources that help your 4- to 6-year-old manage their emotions in challenging moments. This toolbox becomes their go-to safe space when they're feeling overwhelmed, anxious, or just need some extra comfort. Tailoring its contents to their specific needs and preferences makes it much more effective.

WHAT TO INCLUDE IN YOUR CALMING TOOLBOX

- Sensory toys: Sensory toys can provide calming input and help them refocus. Items like fidget spinners, squishy stress balls, textured balls, or sensory bottles filled with glitter and water are great options. Experiment with different types to see what resonates best with your little one.
- Emotions charts: Creating an emotions chart can be helpful. Include various faces representing different emotions (happy, sad, angry, anxious, etc.), and have them point to the face that reflects how they feel. This visual aid makes it easier for your child to identify and communicate their emotions.
- Visuals and social stories: Consider adding visuals that

outline calming strategies. These could be step-by-step guides with pictures, showing what to do when feeling overwhelmed—like taking deep breaths, squeezing a favorite toy, blowing out imaginary candles, or finding a quiet spot. Social stories explaining calming techniques can also help your 4- to 6-year-old understand when and how to use these strategies.

- Calming music or sounds: If they find comfort in music, consider including a playlist of calming songs or nature sounds. Creating a special "calm" playlist together can make it even more meaningful. Music can be incredibly soothing and provide them with a familiar backdrop during stressful moments.
- Comfort items: Sometimes, the simplest items can be the most effective. Think about including things like a favorite stuffed animal, a soft blanket, or a weighted lap pad. These familiar comforts can help your kid feel secure and grounded.
- Mindfulness tools: Incorporate mindfulness techniques into your toolbox. Include tools like a breathing ball that expands with every inhale and deflates with every exhale. Simple visual prompts for guided breathing exercises can also be helpful, especially for visual learners.

HOW TO USE THE CALMING TOOLBOX

Once you've filled your toolbox, it's time to introduce it to your little one. Start by explaining that this is their special box, filled with tools to help when they're feeling big emotions. Encourage them to explore everything inside and figure out which items make them feel better. Let them know it's okay if different tools work at different times or in different ways.

You can even make it a routine: When your 4- to 6-year-old starts to feel overwhelmed, gently guide them to their toolbox. Encourage them to choose an item they think will help. This not only empowers them to take charge of their emotions but also reinforces their ability to manage their feelings and self-regulate consistently over time.

Building a calming toolbox is just one of many ways to support your child's emotional development. Remember, it's okay to try different strategies and adjust as you learn what works best for them. You're learning and growing alongside them, and every small step counts.

As you work on this, don't forget to take care of yourself, too. Parenting can be challenging, but your strength and resilience make a huge difference. Lean on your support network, share your experiences, and celebrate all the wins along the way. You're doing great, and your love and dedication are the foundation of your little one's emotional growth.

IMPLEMENTING POSITIVE REINFORCEMENT DURING MELTDOWNS

Studies show that positive reinforcement is a powerful tool for guiding 4- to 6-year-old children toward better emotional regulation, especially during challenging moments. This approach focuses on rewarding good behaviors to encourage them, rather than punishing negative actions (Mazefsky et al., 2013). Let's talk about some ways you can use this approach to handle emotional eruptions more easily.

Reinforce your young learner's calm behavior through specific praise, such as saying, "I noticed how you took deep breaths to calm down—that was great!" to help them understand and repeat positive actions. Additionally, consider creating a reward system, like a sticker chart, where they earn stickers for managing frustration with words. Once they accumulate enough stickers, offer a reward, such as choosing a family activity or receiving a small toy. Aim for rewards that align with their interests to keep them engaged and motivated.

Celebrating all of their wins is imperative in promoting a growth mindset. They benefit from regular reminders of their abilities and successes, particularly when facing emotional challenges. Each small step they take toward managing their emotions is a milestone worth celebrating. For example, when they communicate a feeling without having a tantrum for the first time, cheer them on with positive words like, "I'm so proud of you for telling me how you feel!" These celebrations strengthen their connection between emotional regulation and positive outcomes.

During moments of emotional distress, use a soothing tone and show patience with your 4- to 6-year-old to model how to handle stress properly. Your gentle presence provides comfort, and helping them label their emotions shows support during tough times.

Consistency and transparency are key—reward specific behaviors regularly and explain your expectations clearly. As they grow, adjust reinforcement strategies to suit their evolving needs. Incorporating these practices into predictable routines, like a sticker chart during morning or bedtime, helps reinforce positive behaviors and fosters emotional regulation.

FINAL INSIGHTS

Understanding and managing emotional meltdowns can feel unbearable at times as a parent, especially when handling the complexities of raising your 4- to 6-year-old on the autism spectrum—which is a totally different ballpark. This chapter serves as your roadmap to recognizing the early signs of emotional dysregulation, helping you minimize the frequency and intensity of these episodes. Identifying specific triggers and observing changes in their body language or facial expressions allows you to step in early and use effective calming strategies. Collaborating with caregivers or professionals can also provide valuable insights and tools to refine your approach.

Remember, by investing time in developing these techniques and emotional regulation strategies, you're not only addressing immediate concerns but also laying the foundation for your child's long-term emotional resilience.

In the next chapter, we'll explore ways to boost communication skills through play—We're getting to the fun stuff now!

KEY TAKEAWAYS

- **Recognize early signs:** Spot physical cues and emotional triggers to intervene early. Look for signs like clenched fists, avoidance behaviors, or changes in tone.
- **Empower with language:** Teach simple emotion words like "mad" or "sad" using tools like charts or flashcards. Practice these words during calm moments to reinforce understanding.
- **Create a calming toolbox:** Personalize a kit filled with sensory toys, comfort items, and mindfulness tools. Include items like noise-canceling headphones or a favorite stuffed toy for immediate comfort.
- **Implement positive reinforcement:** Celebrate successes to encourage self-regulation and confidence. For instance, praise their use of calming strategies with phrases like, "I'm proud of how you stayed calm."
- **Build a supportive environment:** Respond with patience, compassion, and consistency to foster emotional growth. Use predictable routines and engage in calming activities together, like deep breathing or reading.

4

BOOSTING COMMUNICATION SKILLS THROUGH PLAY

Boosting your 4- to 6-year-old's communication skills can be both fun and effective through play. By weaving playful strategies into your daily routines, you'll create an environment where communication naturally flourishes. Everyday activities and favorite characters can become opportunities for practicing language and understanding nonverbal cues. Engaging in this way not only nurtures their growing communication abilities but also deepens your relationship.

In this chapter, we'll venture into a variety of play-based strategies to boost verbal and nonverbal communication skills. We'll discuss how role-playing games expand vocabulary and encourage conversational practice. Let's throw extra emphasis on keeping the process engaging and catering it to their unique preferences, so you can maintain a supportive environment where your little one feels confident expressing themselves.

Role-Playing Games to Foster Language Development

Incorporating role-playing activities into your daily routines offers a powerful way to build communication skills. These playful scenarios create an environment where language development unfolds naturally and effectively. Let's explore practical ways to use role-playing to unlock your 4- to 6-year-old's communication superpowers.

Turn everyday activities, like grocery shopping, into role-playing adventures. Encourage them to request items, describe products, or pretend to play the cashier. This helps your child practice taking turns and applying language in real-life ways. Adding their favorite characters from books, movies, or TV shows can make these sessions even more engaging. Imitating familiar dialogue can help them practice emotional expression and recognition of social cues. By combining real-world experiences with favorite characters, your young learner can strengthen their social language skills and develop a deeper understanding of emotions.

To make these play sessions even more valuable, integrate props and costumes. You don't need to invest in elaborate outfits; simple household items can serve as excellent tools for imagination. A spoon might become a microphone, or a towel draped over their shoulders could turn into a superhero cape. These tactile elements support verbal communication by offering physical prompts that stimulate dialogue. Props and costumes also encourage deeper engagement with the scenario, prompting your little one to narrate their actions or describe the props in detail, which helps expand their vocabulary.

It's also crucial to set specific communication goals during these role-play activities. Think about what aspects of communication you would like to improve in your child. Whether it's building vocabulary, strengthening sentence structure, or learning to take turns speaking, clearly defining these goals beforehand helps you tailor the session to meet those objectives. For instance, if one goal is to build vocabulary, focus on using and explaining new words related to the chosen scenario. If the objective is to improve conversational flow, engage in back-and-forth exchanges by asking and answering questions within the role-play context. Setting clear targets helps structure your interactions and provides a benchmark to track progress.

As you embark on these fun little adventures together, remember that consistency is key. Regularly scheduled role-playing sessions offer amazing benefits for your child's communication skills. Over time, you'll likely see improvements not just in their ability to use language but also in their confidence to interact socially. The goal is to create a supportive environment where they feel safe and motivated to explore language at their own pace.

Real Life Story: Agatha and Her Parents

When Agatha, who was 4 years old, was diagnosed with autism, her parents noticed that she got anxious whenever it was time for a doctor's appointment. Their normally lively little girl, who loved spending hours playing with her toys, would shut down the moment they mentioned the doctor's office. To help her feel more comfortable, they decided to turn her favorite activity, playing, into a solution.

They bought her a doctor's kit, a tiny lab coat, and a toy stethoscope. Soon enough, their living room became Agatha's clinic. Family members took turns as her patient, even bringing her cherished teddy bear into the "waiting room."

At first, Agatha was hesitant, mimicking what she had seen at the doctor's office but speaking very few words. However, as the family continued to play, her confidence began to grow. She started using new words—like "doctor" and "checkup"—and her enthusiasm for the game became evident.

Agatha's role-playing time with her family didn't just help her language development; it transformed her experience with doctor visits. Now, she eagerly talks about being brave, like her teddy bear, during her own appointments. For her parents, watching her blossom into a little doctor during playtime served as a beautiful reminder that growth thrives in playful and supportive environments.

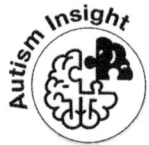

Visual Aids to Improve Nonverbal INTERACTION

Utilizing visual supports can greatly improve your little one's ability to understand and express themselves. As a parent, you might wonder how to effectively support communication for your little one on the autism spectrum. Here's how visual tools can help build nonverbal communication skills.

PICTURE EXCHANGE COMMUNICATION SYSTEMS (PECS)

This is an innovative tool designed specifically to support effective nonverbal communication for your child. PECS sets the foundation by using pictures or symbols that allow them to express their needs, wants, and thoughts without relying solely on spoken language (Picture Exchange Communication System (PECS), 2024). Think of it as a toolkit where each picture becomes a tool they can use to convey a message or start a conversation.

This exchange isn't just about communicating desires; it broadens their ability to interact with the world around them and builds meaningful relationships with caregivers and peers. By integrating PECS, you provide a sense of autonomy, empowering your little one to make choices and express their emotions clearly.

When implementing PECS, personalization is key. Start

with pictures of familiar objects or favorite activities to keep your child engaged and motivated. The process of exchanging a picture to communicate can initially feel novel, but with patience and practice, it becomes a natural part of their vocabulary. To ensure the system stays relevant and engaging, regularly update the set of pictures as they grow and their interests evolve.

VISUAL SCHEDULES

Visual schedules are invaluable for outlining daily routines and reducing anxiety in your 4- to 6-year-old by providing a clear, predictable structure. By using images or symbols, these schedules help them anticipate tasks and transitions, such as waking up, brushing their teeth, or getting dressed, which creates a sense of comfort.

As your son or daughter becomes familiar with the schedule, it promotes independence, allowing them to manage their day with minimal adult guidance. Start with a few activities and gradually expand as they become more comfortable. Visual schedules encourage active participation and confidence, and praising their progress sends signals to their growing brains, letting them know that these behaviors are good behaviors.

GESTURE CARDS

Using gesture cards adds another dimension to understanding and expressing emotions and actions. These cards depict common gestures, such as waving or smiling, along with emotions like happiness or frustration.

They serve as visual prompts to help your kid attach specific feelings or actions to the correct gestures, strengthening both comprehension and expression. To introduce gesture cards, show one card at a time, model the gesture yourself, and encourage your young learner to imitate it.

This interactive method turns learning into an engaging activity rather than just another task, building a strong foundation for effective nonverbal communication.

STORYTELLING FOR NONVERBAL CUES

Storytelling offers another great resource for teaching appropriate nonverbal cues and social expectations. By breaking down everyday social situations into simple narratives, storytelling helps your child understand body language, facial expressions, and other nonverbal signals.

Focus on specific scenarios that are relevant to their daily life. For example, point out in a story someone who's greeting a friend at school or sharing toys—and depict the necessary cues involved in those interactions.

Setting Aside Intentional Playtime for Communication Practice

Boosting your 4- to 6-year-old's communication skills can be a heck of a ride, let me tell you! One helpful tip is to weave play into your daily routines, allowing it to serve as both a learning experience and a developmental tool. Doing this allows them to build verbal and nonverbal communication while supporting their broader growth and development.

To start, establish a designated communication time. This structured period focuses on activities specifically designed to brighten their communication skills. Setting aside time each day dedicated solely to communication through play establishes consistency and helps build a reliable routine. It helps distinguish this time from free play, emphasizing its importance and making both you and your young learner more focused on communication objectives during these sessions.

Your dedicated playtime should include carefully selected

and engaging activities that naturally inspire conversation. Consider games involving turn-taking, storytelling, or simple board games that require interaction. These activities should be enjoyable for your child, motivating them to participate willingly and enthusiastically. The goal is to make communication an appealing task rather than a forced activity. By selecting a fun yet instructive mix of games, you create an environment where learning feels like play.

Use open-ended questions during playtime to stimulate your young learner's critical thinking and encourage deeper conversations. These questions don't have a correct answer, allowing them to think creatively and express themselves more freely. Instead of asking, "Is this block red?" which requires a simple yes or no answer, ask, "What else can we build with these blocks?" Open-ended questions are more beneficial, as they promote broader language use and help your bright adventurer share their ideas and emotions. This approach fosters dialogue, expands vocabulary, and boosts confidence.

Modeling effective communication is imperative for nurturing communication skills through play. Demonstrate appropriate social etiquette and conversational behaviors, such as making eye contact, taking turns speaking, and using polite greetings. During play, narrating your actions or thoughts provides clear examples and reinforces the social cues and language structures you want them to emulate. For instance, while playing a game, say, "I'm so excited to play this with you! Now it's your turn. What do you want to play next?" By modeling enthusiasm and proper speech patterns, you encourage your little one to mimic these interactions in their own communications.

Expressing emotions and appreciation, such as thanking and hugging, can also be integrated into playtime. These simple gestures are powerful tools for teaching empathy and emotional expression. After playing together, say, "I had so much fun building this with you. Thank you for playing with me! May I give you a hug?" These expressions validate your child's feelings while encouraging them to acknowledge others' emotions positively. Moreover, physical gestures like hugs can reinforce verbal messages and help them understand the connection between words and emotions. Teaching them to ask permission regarding physical gestures helps them feel safe within their own personal space and helps them understand the importance of respecting others' boundaries.

Providing opportunities to engage all five senses during play can also build their communication skills. Activities that incorporate sight, sound, touch, smell, and taste create varied experiences that prompt different reactions and interactions. Something like a sensory bin filled with colorful objects, fragrant playdough, or textured materials can be an excellent tool for discussion. Encourage them to describe what they see, feel, or smell, which promotes the use of descriptive language. This leads to an expanded vocabulary and enhanced expressive capabilities.

Play isn't just about having fun; it provides a foundation for future learning and life skills development. Through both structured and unstructured play, your child learns by trying things, comparing results, asking questions, and meeting challenges. They develop confidence and curiosity, as well as the ability to plan, organize, and make decisions. These skills are needed for effective communication.

COLLABORATION TIPS FOR UNIFIED COMMUNICATION STRATEGIES

When helping your 4- to 6-year-old on the autism spectrum build their communication skills, a collaborative approach can be incredibly effective. Team up with educators and caregivers to ensure a consistent framework that supports their growth and language development. Everyone involved must be on the same page, sharing communication goals and strategies.

Start by setting clear communication objectives and discussing them with everyone involved. When the goals are effectively communicated to caregivers and educators, they can consistently reinforce them in various activities and environments. For instance, if one of the goals is to encourage more verbal interaction, the same approach can be applied during classroom activities, playdates, and at home, making sure your learner receives a unified message about what's expected and encouraged.

Consistency across different environments is key to solidifying learned communication behaviors. Being on the autism spectrum, your young learner often excels with routine and predictability, so when caregivers and educators use similar language cues and reinforcement strategies, it creates a stable learning environment. This might mean using the same phrases for greetings, employing identical prompts for requesting items, or maintaining consistent responses to their attempts at communication. With a little consistency, they will eventually understand that the same rules apply everywhere, creating phenomenal communication skills.

Utilizing shared resources like journals or progress charts is also effective. These tools track improvements, identify challenges, and provide a comprehensive record of your kiddo's progress. Caregivers and educators can jot down observations, strategies that work well, and areas needing more focus. Regularly sharing these records means that everyone is on the same page and goals for communication are front and center.

Creating a strong team of champions who are always rooting for your little one will play a huge role in their success with communication later on. This team may consist of family, teachers, even neighbors—the more the merrier! Open lines of communication allow for the exchange of ideas and experiences, paving the way for tailored strategies that cater to your child's specific needs. Family members might notice behaviors or triggers at home that educators may not see, while teachers can share valuable observations from classroom settings that are beneficial at home. Working together and sharing these insights helps both sides develop a deeper understanding of your young learner's strengths and areas for growth, leading to a more robust support systems.

FINAL INSIGHTS

In this chapter, we've covered the power of role-playing and visual aids in strengthening your 4- to 6-year-old's communication skills. Transforming everyday scenarios, such as preparing for a visit to the doctor or shopping, into playful role-playing opportunities helps them learn words while understanding social nuances and emotions.

Setting aside dedicated playtime is also pivotal in their communication development. By using tools like PECS cards and gesture charts, and making communication practice a fun and consistent part of your routine, you nurture your young learner's expressive abilities in a safe and supportive environment.

KEY TAKEAWAYS

- **Role-playing is a powerful tool:** Use scenarios like grocery shopping or preparing for bedtime to encourage communication, interaction, and growth.
- **Incorporating favorite toys eases anxiety:** Pair their favorite toys with tools like PECS cards or gesture charts to simplify nonverbal communication and make interactions more engaging.
- **Family involvement fosters connection:** Use structured playtime for activities like pretend cooking or storytelling, where siblings or caregivers can participate to enhance language development and deepen family bonds.
- **Repetition builds confidence:** Consistent practice helps your young learner feel secure and motivated to express themselves.
- **Play is more than fun; it's therapeutic:** Structured play not only reduces anxiety but also builds essential skills in a supportive environment.

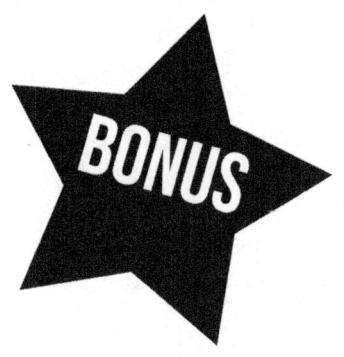

PRINTABLE PECS CARDS FOR YOUR 4- TO 6-YEAR-OLD ON THE AUTISM SPECTRUM

Communication is a powerful tool, and I'm thrilled to share this exclusive bonus: a professionally designed set of **35 Printable PECS (Picture Exchange Communication System) cards** tailored for your child aged 4-6 on the autism spectrum. These cards are designed to help your young learner express themselves, navigate routines, and better understand their emotions and needs.

This bonus provides a professionally formatted, high-resolution PDF, ready for easy and cost-effective printing, so you can start using them right away!

HOW THESE PECS CARDS CAN HELP

In this set, you'll find visually engaging cards to help your child:

- **Communicate Daily Routines**: Examples include brushing teeth, getting dressed, and eating breakfast.
- **Express Basic Needs**: Cards like "I'm hungry," "I need help," and "I'm thirsty."
- **Understand Emotions and Feelings**: Cards for happy, sad, tired, and more.

- **Enjoy Play and Activities**: Examples include playing ball, coloring, and reading.
- **Navigate Sensory Needs**: Cards for "too loud," "calm time," and "it's too bright."
- **Learn in Fun Ways**: Numbers, shapes, colors, and more.

With these cards, your child will have the tools to express their needs, navigate transitions, and build confidence in communication.

HOW TO CLAIM YOUR FREE PECS CARDS

It's easy to get started:

1. **Visit the Website**: Go to https://www.parentingmastery series.com/autism-resource1 or scan the QR code below.

2. **Download the PDF**: Instantly access your printable cards, organized into categories for convenience.

3. **Print and Use:** Print the cards and begin using them to support your child's communication journey.

These PECS cards are thoughtfully designed to foster communication, independence, and emotional growth in your child. By integrating them into your daily routines, you can create a more supportive and engaging environment for your little one.

SCAN HERE TO ACCESS YOUR FREE PECS CARDS

Warmly, Heather

SOCIAL SKILLS FOR LIFE

Social skills are crucial for managing relationships and navigating the world, including interactions with family, friends, and peers. For a parent of a 4- to 6-year-old on the autism spectrum, teaching these skills can seem challenging. You may find yourself wondering how to best support their social development in a way that feels both effective and engaging.

Introducing structured play activities focused on empathy and turn-taking offers a valuable way to support their growth. These strategies create pathways for your little one to relate to others, building their confidence and ability to navigate those tricky social situations.

This chapter provides practical ways to incorporate empathy-building exercises and simple games into your child's routine to enrich their social life. By integrating playful strategies into daily routines, this journey can become both manageable and enjoyable for you and your child.

Creating Opportunities for Role-Play to Practice Empathy

Role-play is a powerful tool for both you and your 4- to 6-year-old to understand and practice empathetic behaviors. When you immerse your kid in relatable scenarios, they gain valuable opportunities to manage complex social situations and develop essential emotional skills. Here are some ways to use role-play to help your little one build empathy.

Start by identifying characters and scenarios that reflect your child's everyday interactions. Choose familiar situations they encounter at home or school, like sharing toys or taking turns on the playground. This approach allows them to explore emotions and responses they might face in real life. When they take on the roles of various characters, your child learns to relate to diverse perspectives, helping them build emotional intelligence. This practice enhances their understanding of how their actions affect others' feelings, which is essential for developing empathy.

For instance, you might role-play a scenario where your child accidentally knocks over another child's block tower. Through guided play, discuss how each character might feel, what they could say to resolve the situation, and how to offer comfort. This type of reflection deepens their understanding of empathy.

Using puppets or dolls in role-playing offers a safe way for your little one to express emotions and practice empathy without the pressure of direct interactions. This creative play allows them to act out scenarios, explore different resolutions, and rehearse social skills in a controlled setting. After role-play, structured discussions with open-ended questions like, "How do you think the character felt?" reinforce empathy by prompting your 4-to 6-year-old to reflect on emotions and social situations, helping deepen their understanding.

Consider each role-play session as a storytelling moment. Ask your son or daughter to explain what their character experienced and reflect on how they solved any challenges they faced. This narrative exercise encourages them to articulate their thoughts and feelings, boosting their ability to empathize with others. Additionally, these discussions provide a chance for you to introduce vocabulary related to emotions, such as "happy," "sad," "frustrated," or "proud," supporting them in building a strong emotional language for expressing themselves and understanding others.

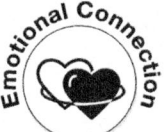

Encouraging peer interactions through playdates is another vital aspect of fostering empathy through role-play. Playdates give your 4- to 6-year-old the opportunity to engage in real-world social scenarios, helping them practice empathy and develop skills like cooperation and communication. When they participate in role-play activities with friends, they not only learn to apply empathy but also develop other social skills, like cooperation and communication. These interactions make the empathy they develop during play more relevant to everyday situations.

Setting up playdates can be exciting for both you and your child. Plan events where children work together to solve problems, such as building a bridge with blocks or creating a pretend community with puppets and dollhouses. These activities encourage teamwork and mutual support. As a parent, actively participating by guiding interactions and gently prompting discussions about feelings and conflict resolution is essential.

Post-play discussion is equally important. Create a calm and supportive environment where your little one feels comfortable reflecting on their experiences. Ask open-ended questions, listen attentively to their responses, and provide gentle feedback to guide their understanding. Encouraging your child to consider alternative outcomes or discuss how different actions could lead to different emotional results reinforces the empathy lessons from role-play.

By doing this, you're helping them naturally internalize empathy and develop meaningful connections with others.

SIMPLE BOARD GAMES FOR LEARNING HOW TO TAKE TURNS

Board games can be a delightful way to teach necessary social skills like turn-taking and patience. Among the hustle and bustle of daily life, these fun activities offer meaningful opportunities for your 4- to 6-year-old to practice and learn. For example, setting up a Candy Land board in front of them lays the foundation for an engaging and educational experience.

Choosing the right game is a key ingredient to throw into the mix—it creates excitement and holds more value. Your young learner has unique interests and is at a specific developmental stage, so choose games wisely, with straightforward, age-appropriate rules being most important. Consider a simple matching game like Guess Who—a game of this nature has less going on, making it much easier to keep stress at bay. When they are interested and actively participating, they tend to grasp these lessons more quickly and authentically.

The importance of structure and clarity cannot be overstated, especially for a child on the autism spectrum. Establishing clear rules before starting ensures everyone understands expectations, and it's smooth sailing after that. Visual aids, like cards with game steps or written instructions in simple language, can minimize confusion and help your child follow along.

As you play, act as a role model for patience, fairness, and sportsmanship. Your 4- to 6-year-old is an absorbent little sponge waiting to see how you respond in any given scenario. Modeling patience and enjoyment during board games provides an example of ideal social behaviors. Displaying positive reactions, whether you win or lose, fosters a healthy mindset in your learner. It helps create a positive association with social interactions, showing them that playing with others can be a fun experience regardless of the outcome.

Creating a routine around board games serves as another layer of reinforcement. Regular game nights, for instance, can offer predictability—a comforting factor for many kids with autism. Knowing that every Friday night involves a round of Chutes and Ladders contributes to a stable environment. This routine reduces anxiety and promotes a sense of security and bonding among family members. Over time, your 4- to 6-year-old will begin to see these sessions not as rigid lessons but as part of their everyday, enjoyable activities that teach important social lessons naturally.

When you engage in these structured yet entertaining activities, your child learns more than just the mechanics of a game. They begin to respect turns, wait patiently, and even strategize about how to approach their next move—all while in the embrace of a supportive, fun atmosphere. These experiences also teach them how to handle frustration when the game doesn't go their way and how to celebrate gracefully, both of which are instrumental for emotional development.

Incremental Complexity in Social Interactions

Understanding how a young learner's social skills develop is important, particularly when you have a child navigating the autism spectrum. Gradually increasing the complexity of social interactions helps strengthen their social development while minimizing stress.

First things first—you need to assess your child's current skills which sets the foundation for developing an effective, personalized strategy. This step allows your approach to mold to their specific needs. Understanding what they can currently do helps you design activities that are appropriately challenging—neither too easy nor too difficult. For example, if your little one can successfully engage in one-on-one playdates, they might be ready for small group settings. This assessment serves as a compass, directing you toward achievable goals while maintaining their sense of security.

Introducing small group activities is a pivotal next step. Small groups provide an ideal environment for nurturing social interactions. These settings are typically less intimidating than larger gatherings, allowing your little explored to practice social skills such as sharing, taking turns, and cooperating with others. For example, a simple game of building blocks with a few peers offers valuable learning opportunities. As they engage with others, your 4- to 6-year-old begins to understand different social roles and expectations in a controlled, supportive atmosphere. Success in these smaller interactions builds confidence and acts as a stepping stone to more significant challenges.

As they become more comfortable and adept at handling small groups, the next level involves expanding their exposure to larger settings. This progression should be gradual. Start by attending larger family gatherings or community events with careful preparation. Use role-playing strategies from the last chapter. Walk through some pretend scenarios with them so they know what to expect. Bring along familiar items to provide comfort in unfamiliar environments. With each new situation tackled and overcome, your learner gains not only new social skills but also an increased sense of confidence.

Placing them in these little stories prepares them for new experiences. These stories are tailored narratives that depict common social scenarios, outlining behavioral expectations and the dynamics involved. They serve as a rehearsal tool, enabling them to visualize and mentally prepare for real-life social challenges. For instance, reading a social story about visiting a playground can help them anticipate what may happen, the roles they might play, and various positive outcomes. Equipped with these insights, your 4- to 6-year-old may feel more confident and less anxious about the unknown.

Developing social cognition, which includes understanding others' intentions and emotions, is another important piece of the puzzle. According to studies, children begin honing these skills quite early on. Their natural preference for movements like eye contact and imitation reflects the foundation of their social capacities (Soto-Icaza et al., 2015). By recognizing and nurturing these emerging abilities, you can support your child's natural inclination to improve their social interactions.

It's important to be patient throughout this process. Like any learning experience, some days will be a slam dunk, others will be a long shot, to say the least. Progress often happens in small steps, and setbacks should be expected. Celebrating milestones, such as your little one initiating a greeting or playing alongside others, encourages their continued effort and reinforces positive behaviors.

As you manage these developments, remember the value of structured discussions after social activities. Including your child in conversations about their experiences promotes reflection. You might ask questions like, "How did you feel when we went to the park today?" or "What did you enjoy most about playing with your friends?" These dialogues deepen their understanding of social scenarios and emotions, reinforcing important lessons learned through interaction.

Creating a Social Skills Checklist

Creating a social skills checklist can be a wonderful way to help you feel more confident in tracking your 4- to 6-year-old's progress while celebrating those victories that often go unnoticed. Social skills like empathy, sharing, turn-taking, and understanding social cues can feel overwhelming to teach, but dividing them into simple, trackable actions provides clarity and gives a sense of hope.

SOCIAL SKILLS CHECKLIST EXAMPLE

- Empathy: Recognize when someone is upset and provide comfort (e.g., offering a hug, toy, or kind words).
- Sharing: Offer a toy during playtime and maintain sharing for at least five minutes.
- Turn-taking: Wait patiently for a turn during a game, demonstrating an understanding of the rules.
- Understanding social cues: Identify when a friend is happy or upset by observing facial expressions or other nonverbal signals.

How it works: Each time your little one completes one of these actions, you check it off. You can even add small rewards or words of encouragement to motivate them, like, "You shared your toy! High-five!" Acknowledging these achievements boosts their confidence and reassures you that they're making progress.

REAL LIFE STORY: SARAH AND HER SON LIAM

Meet Sarah and her son, Liam. At 4 years old, Liam was diagnosed with autism, and Sarah often felt overwhelmed as she tried to help him connect with other kids. Simple things like sharing or recognizing when someone was upset felt like significant challenges.

After learning about social skills checklists, Sarah decided to create one with a few simple goals: sharing toys with friends, waiting for Liam's turn during games, and understanding when someone was sad or upset. She added small, clear tasks that Liam could accomplish, and they used stickers with smiley faces to mark his progress.

At first, the steps seemed slow—Liam didn't always understand why sharing was important. But after a few weeks, Sarah noticed Liam offering his toy without being asked. Then, during playtime, he waited for his turn without frustration, and eventually, he even brought a toy to comfort a friend who was crying.

Sarah felt like these small victories were monumental. Having the checklist allowed her to track progress and see that Liam was learning and growing, even if it wasn't always obvious on a daily basis. And most importantly, it gave her something concrete to celebrate with her son.

Creating your own checklist allows you to focus on what matters most—progress, no matter how small, is still progress. It also gives you tangible opportunities to celebrate your little one's achievements, boosting their confidence and reinforcing your reassurance throughout the process.

FINAL INSIGHTS

In this chapter, we've gone over how structured play can help your 4- to 6-year-old develop empathy and learn turn-taking. By utilizing tools like role-play and board games, you create an engaging learning environment where they can explore and understand emotions in a safe and controlled setting. Incorporating familiar scenarios into role-playing activities, like preparing for a visit to the doctor or sharing toys, lets your child step into different roles. This helps them see how their actions impact others' feelings.

Additionally, simple board games, like Candy Land or Connect 4, become a gateway for teaching valuable social skills like patience, cooperation, and turn-taking—all while having fun. Regularly playing these games fosters routines that encourage your learner to practice these skills while enjoying meaningful time with family.

This chapter serves as a reminder that with the right tools and guidance, nurturing these vital skills isn't only possible but also immensely rewarding for both you and your loved one. In the next chapter, I think it's important that we talk about practical strategies to help your young learner transition smoothly into a school environment.

KEY TAKEAWAYS

- **Structured play and empathy-building exercises:** Introducing role-play, such as sharing toys or taking turns, helps teach empathy and essential social skills.
- **Role-playing to teach empathy:** Familiar situations, like visiting the doctor, let your 4- to 6-year-old step into others' shoes and understand how their actions impact others.
- **Using tools such as puppets and dolls:** Puppets or dolls can help your child express emotions and experiment with social responses. For example, acting out a scenario where a puppet shares a toy encourages turn-taking and empathy.
- **The value of post-play discussions:** After role-playing or playdates, sit with your little one to reflect. Ask questions like, "How do you think the other person felt?" or "What could we do differently next time?" to encourage emotional understanding.

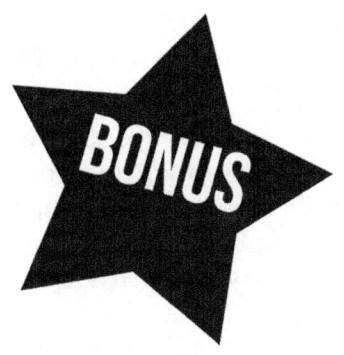

I'm so excited to share something special with you: **SPARK Adventures—Audio Short Stories for Your 4- to 6-year-old.** These stories are filled with fun, adventure, and important lessons like kindness, courage, and problem-solving. They're designed to inspire young minds and make story time a magical part of your routine.

This collection features five professionally narrated stories tailored specifically for your child on the autism spectrum, aged 4 to 6. You can choose one story to enjoy with your little one—completely free.

HOW TO GET YOUR FREE STORY

It's easy to get started:

1. **Visit the Website**: Go to https://www.ParentingMastery Series.com/Autism/AdventureSeriesAudio or scan the QR code on the next page.

2. **Choose a Story**: Pick your 4- to 6-year-old's favorite adventure from the dropdown menu.

3. **Listen and Enjoy**: Download your story as an MP3 and play it during quiet time, bedtime, or whenever they need a spark of imagination.

WHY SPARK ADVENTURES?

These stories are crafted to captivate your little learner's imagination while gently introducing life lessons in a way that's fun and engaging. With professional narration and age-appropriate themes, they're the perfect way to nurture creativity and growth at this important stage.

Take a moment to explore the website and find the perfect story for your child. It's a small way to bring even more joy and inspiration into their day.

SCAN HERE TO CLAIM YOUR FREE STORY

Warmly, Heather

SCHOOL READINESS

Studies continue to show that children on the autism spectrum often face significant challenges when starting school, especially with social interactions (Marsh et al., 2017). Preparing your 4- to 6-year-old for school requires thoughtful planning, support, and patience. As you begin this process, it's important to create an environment that mimics the school setting to help make the transition smoother and less chaotic. You'll find that establishing routines at home similar to those they will experience in school helps your young learner feel more confident and comfortable with the impending changes. Starting these school-like habits early equips them with the tools to approach this new stage in their life with excitement rather than fear.

In this chapter, we'll explore practical strategies that can make a world of difference as your little one prepares for school. We'll focus on how establishing structured routines at home can simplify transitions, ensuring that both you and your little one feel prepared for the journey ahead.

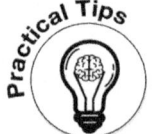 ## Developing a School-Like Routine at Home

Studies show that establishing a structured home routine that mirrors school expectations can greatly ease the transition for your 4- to 6-year-old on the autism spectrum (Ibañez et al., 2018). For you as a parent, creating this environment is an essential step in preparing your young learner to adapt to the school's structured schedule and routines. Implementing these strategies at home can help your child build familiarity and confidence.

Teaching the importance of school start times may be a little rocky at first, but your 4- to 6-year-old will get the hang of it in no time. You can begin establishing a morning schedule at home to align with the typical school day. Start by waking your son or daughter up at the same time they would need to wake up for school. Gradually adjust bedtime to make sure they get adequate rest, making wake-up time easier. In the mornings, replicate the school's pre-start routine by getting dressed, having breakfast, and packing a bag—even if it's just a symbolic exercise with chosen items. This consistent practice reinforces the morning routine, sets clear expectations, and helps make it a natural habit for your child.

Using visual schedules to establish predictability within their daily routine works wonders. Visual cards can serve as excellent tools. These visuals guide your little one through each step in sequence—from brushing their teeth to putting away toys. The use of images helps them associate specific activities with time blocks, assisting them in understanding what comes next. Regularly update and review these visual schedules, allowing your learner to become more comfortable and independent in managing their time.

Incorporating visual timers can further improve their time management skills. These timers provide a clear indicator of how much time remains for an activity before transitioning to the next. One thing you could do is set a timer during playtime or when doing a simple chore. The visible nature of a countdown clock offers your 4- to 6-year-old an understanding of elapsed time without relying solely on numerical concepts, which might be challenging for their young mind. Over time, your little one can learn to internalize these cues, helping them develop a more intuitive grasp of time management.

To support social readiness, introduce role-playing scenarios to simulate expected school interactions. These activities give your child the chance to rehearse common social situations they might encounter at school. Create simple scripts for interactions, like greeting a teacher, joining a group activity, or asking for help. As you act out these scenarios together, emphasize the importance of eye contact, turn-taking, and polite communication. Encourage them to express themselves and react naturally, helping them build confidence and social awareness.

Practicing Separation and Aligning Expectations

Transitioning your young learner on the autism spectrum to school can be an emotional journey, both for you and them. One of the key steps in this transition is helping them feel comfortable with separation from caregivers and gain a better understanding of what to expect from the school environment. This involves easing separation anxiety through gradual exposure and thoughtful preparation.

Start by introducing short separations as practice for the school drop-off scenario. Taking this small step helps your little adventurer build confidence, showing them that being apart from you is temporary and nothing to fear. Begin by leaving them with a familiar family member or friend for brief periods, gradually increasing the duration over time. This process not only allows your learner to understand that you'll always return but also begins to normalize the concept of spending time apart.

Discussing school expectations with your 4- to 6-year-old helps reduce fear and build excitement for this new stage. They may often fear the unknown, so providing information about what will happen at school can be reassuring. Explain daily routines they might encounter, such as snack times, play sessions, and lessons, using simple language they can easily grasp. Storytelling or reading books about starting school provides relatable scenarios that demonstrate a typical day, making the experience feel more concrete and less scary. Engage them in conversations about school activities, allowing them to express their feelings, ask questions, and share any concerns. This dialogue can help transform apprehension into anticipation.

Comfort objects are another valuable tool in easing initial separation anxiety. Allow your little one to bring a favorite item from home, such as a blanket or teddy bear, to school. These objects provide a tangible link to home and serve as a soothing reminder during moments of unease. Although it may seem like a small act, bringing a familiar item from home can boost their mood and make them feel safe.

Celebrating successes and reinforcing positive outcomes are essential to nurturing their resilience and self-confidence through these transitions. Each successful separation, no matter how minor, offers an opportunity to celebrate progress. Recognize and praise your learner's courage in managing goodbyes and accepting new environments. You might choose to recognize these accomplishments with verbal affirmations, stickers, or a small reward, all of which can further motivate them to embrace future challenges with enthusiasm.

Using these strategies as a part of your plan requires patience and consistency. It's a gradual process where every step forward fosters greater adaptability in your child. Remember, your positive reinforcement and unwavering belief in their ability to handle this change make all the difference. Rely on your support system and collaborate with teachers who can offer additional reassurance during these critical moments. When you work together as a team, you create an inclusive and welcoming atmosphere that encourages your little one to shine.

Throughout this process, remember that your child's comfort level and timeline are unique. If challenges arise, stay flexible and adapt your approach, as necessary. Maintain open communication with educators so everyone is in the loop—this will be a sure way of supporting your 4- to 6-year-old in a way that is specially designed for them.

BUILDING RELATIONSHIPS WITH TEACHING STAFF

Building strong connections with your child's educational staff can greatly ease their transition to school. Establishing these relationships as a parent is essential for creating a supportive and understanding environment tailored to their unique needs. Here are some strategies to help you build these vital connections.

First, arranging introductory meetings with teachers before the school year starts can help foster familiarity. This initial step is more than just small talk, like discussing the weather or joking about the wild things that come out of kids' mouths; it's about allowing both parties—parents and teachers—to share insights into your 4- to 6-year-old's world. Understanding your little learner's preferences, strengths, and challenges allows teachers to prepare effectively. Especially for kids on the autism spectrum, knowing what triggers anxiety or causes discomfort can be invaluable information for the teacher. Use these meetings as an opportunity to discuss how the classroom environment may need to be adjusted to accommodate sensory sensitivities or other specific needs. Proactive discussions like these set a positive tone for collaboration and ensure the teacher knows how to support your child right from the start. Such informational exchanges are supported by the principles of parental engagement, which advocate for active involvement in educational planning (Fernández Cerero, José et al., 2024).

Encouraging classroom visits before school officially begins is another way to reduce fear of the unknown for your little one. A new environment can be intimidating, especially for a child with autism aged 4 to 6 who may thrive on routine and predictability. Allowing them to familiarize themselves with the physical space, meet key staff members beforehand, and even spend short amounts of time playing or engaging in activities there can make all the difference. It's like rehearsing for a big event—the more familiar they are with the setting, the less overwhelming it will appear when school starts for real. These visits can also provide a chance for you to observe how your learner will interact with the environment and identify any areas that might require special accommodations or extra support.

Something else to consider is maintaining open communication between parents and teachers about your 4- to 6-year-old's specific needs. Open lines of communication form the backbone of successful parent-teacher partnerships. Establish preferred methods of regular contact through emails, notes, or scheduled meetings to ensure timely updates on your learner's progress and any immediate concerns that come to the surface.

Communication isn't solely about sharing problems, it's also about recognizing and celebrating successes. Regular chats about daily experiences can provide deeper insights into their social and academic growth. As highlighted by research, consistent dialogue fosters mutual understanding and enriches the support network surrounding your child (Khatab et al., 2024).

Beyond the teacher-parent dynamic, engaging in school events can promote a sense of belonging within the educational community. Participating in activities such as back-to-school nights, family events, or even volunteering opportunities can strengthen your connection with the school's culture and other families. These events offer informal settings where you can meet teachers and staff, gaining insights into the curriculum and the school's ethos. More importantly, your involvement demonstrates to your little one that you're committed to their education and comfortable in the school environment yourself. This shared participation can boost their confidence and comfort within the school setting.

Using Visual and Play-Based Learning Techniques

As we talked about earlier, when preparing your 4- to 6-year-old for the transition to school, using visual aids and play-based methods can create an engaging and less stressful learning environment. Having a visual representation of daily tasks or lesson plans helps them anticipate what comes next, reducing anxiety associated with new or unexpected situations.

Revisiting PECS, consider a morning routine chart as a tool that illustrates each step they need to take before heading to school. For instance, a sequence of pictures might show waking up, brushing teeth, getting dressed, having breakfast, and grabbing a symbolic school bag. Visualizing these steps can turn a potentially chaotic morning into a calm and predictable routine, alleviating stress for you and your little one.

While visual aids lay a foundation, play-based learning mimics real-world experiences that are both cheerful and educational. It combines fun with academic growth, engaging your young learner's natural curiosity and channeling it into productive exploration. In this context, playing becomes an active form of learning where they manipulate objects, solve problems, and make discoveries.

Imagine integrating play-based learning by setting up a "shopping store" at home. Through this activity, your little one can learn numbers and counting. By mirroring classroom activities during play, they can experience a smoother transition between home and school environments, helping to ease their transition.

Beyond structured play, encouraging spontaneous exploration fosters creativity and supports learning experiences similar to those in school. When your little one engages in free play, they'll exercise decision-making skills and boost self-confidence. A backyard nature scavenger hunt can be a thrilling way to teach about plants or insects. These activities provide opportunities for exploration while sprinkling a bit of educational content in the mix.

Providing opportunities for creative play is imperative. Materials like blocks, art supplies, or musical instruments encourage your 4- to 6-year-old to experiment, express themselves, and build narratives. Creative play enhances cognitive development and reflects how learning unfolds in school—by embracing trial, error, and persistence.

Role-playing and games offer another dimension to learning, easing the acquisition of academic and social skills in a stress-free manner. Through role-playing, your child can develop empathy and understanding by seeing situations from others' perspectives. For example, pretending to be a teacher or a classmate can prepare them for classroom interactions, teaching appropriate ways to express thoughts and emotions.

Games structured around rules, such as board games or card games, introduce concepts of fairness, patience, cooperation, and turn-taking—skills critical in a classroom setting. They also provide an opportunity for you, as a parent, to guide your little one in a relaxed and supportive environment. Playing a simple game like "Simon Says" can improve listening skills and the ability to follow directions, laying the groundwork for absorbing classroom instructions.

Through role-play and games, they can develop resilience

by facing challenges within a safe and controlled environment. This type of play supports their ability to manage school-related stress, reinforcing the idea that making mistakes is part of learning and growth. By working through scenarios in their play world, they gain insights that transfer seamlessly into real-life situations.

It's important to remember that structure and flexibility in approach go hand in hand. Providing choices allows your young learner to pursue their interests, fostering deeper engagement and more meaningful learning experiences. Balancing guided activities with freedom of choice respects their autonomy and builds confidence.

Real Life Story: The Jensen Family

The Jensen family has been preparing their five-year-old daughter, Abby, for school with a careful blend of play and practice. Abby, recently diagnosed with autism, thrives on routine, so the family created a daily "school" game at home. Every morning, they set up a small "classroom" with her favorite stuffed animals as classmates, and her older brother, Ethan, acts as the teacher, gently leading her through activities like circle time, snack breaks, and story hour. Together, they practice sitting at a small desk, raising her hand to answer questions, and singing welcoming songs. These playful routines have gradually eased Abby's anxiety, turning school into a familiar and friendly experience rather than a source of fear.

Every Tuesday, the Jensens visit Abby's future classroom while it's still empty, letting her explore freely and become comfortable in the space. She walks the halls, touches the desks, and peeks inside the cubbies, gradually creating a mental map of her new surroundings. After three months of these weekly visits, the school staff arranged brief meetups with a few children from her future class, helping her ease into the social side of things with minimal pressure. For the Jensens, these small steps feel like victories, building confidence in Abby—and in themselves—that she'll soon be ready to take on her school days with joy and ease.

FINAL INSIGHTS

As you move forward with preparing your 4- to 6-year-old for school, remember the importance of building a routine that mirrors school life at home. These steps, though they may seem simple, lay a solid foundation to help them feel more comfortable and confident in making this big transition. This chapter was all about discussing ways to establish predictable daily patterns with your young learner. Whether through visual schedules or timers, these tools enhance their time management skills and understanding of their new environment, while involving the family fosters teamwork in preparing for this transition.

We also revisited the value of role-playing social scenarios, such as greeting teachers or asking for help, to further build school readiness by providing real experiences similar to those they may encounter with educators and peers.

This chapter serves as a reminder that with the right tools and guidance, the school transition can be an exciting journey with so much to look forward to. In the next chapter, we'll explore strategies to nurture your little one's independence and build their confidence for success in school and beyond.

KEY TAKEAWAYS

- **Establish a structured home routine similar to school:** A structured routine mimicking school life helps your 4- to 6-year-old adjust to new expectations.
- **Incorporate visual tools and timers:** Use visual schedules, such as picture charts for morning routines, or countdown timers to create predictability and reduce anxiety during transitions.
- **Prepare for social readiness with role-playing:** Role-play common school scenarios, like raising a hand to answer a question or navigating lunchroom routines, to build confidence in social interactions.
- **Gradually ease separation anxiety:** Practice short separations, like leaving your child with a trusted caregiver for brief periods, and celebrate small wins to build trust and confidence.
- **Build relationships and collaborate with teachers:** Connect with teachers early to share insights about your child's strengths, triggers, and needs. Consider providing a simple handout or summary to ensure they can create a supportive and inclusive environment.

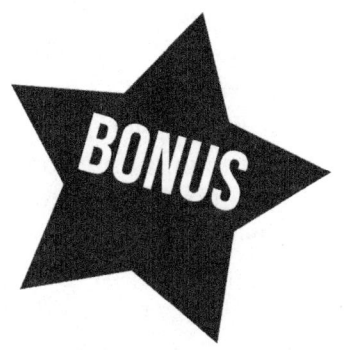

Preparing your child for school requires focus, energy, and emotional stability. Nutrition plays a pivotal role in supporting these areas, which is why I've created this guide, titled **The Ultimate Ketogenic Guide for Your Child on the Autism Spectrum: Tailored for Ages 4–6** as a free downloadable PDF.

This comprehensive guide explores how a ketogenic diet can support their unique needs, helping you make informed nutritional choices that positively impact development.

HOW THIS PDF GUIDE CAN HELP YOUR CHILD

In this guide, you'll discover how a ketogenic diet may benefit your 4- to 6-year-old on the autism spectrum by:

1. **Improving Focus and Behavior**: Stabilizing energy levels for better attention and concentration.

2. **Supporting Emotional Regulation:** Reducing irritability and fostering emotional balance through balanced nutrition.

3. **Simplifying Meal Planning**: Providing easy, kid-friendly recipes designed for your child's age group.

WHY THIS MATTERS?

Research suggests that dietary choices can significantly impact focus, behavior, and overall emotional well-being in children with autism. Whether you're exploring dietary changes or just curious about the connection between nutrition and autism, this guide provides clear and actionable information.

HOW TO DOWNLOAD YOUR FREE PDF GUIDE

Getting your copy is simple!

1. **Visit:** https://www.parentingmasteryseries.com/autism-resource1 to download your free guide, or

2. **Scan the QR code below** to access the PDF instantly:

Warmly, Heather

7
PROMOTING INDEPENDENCE AND CONFIDENCE

Promoting independence and confidence in your 4- to 6-year-old on the autism spectrum is a meaningful and rewarding adventure that begins with creating responsibility through daily tasks, decision-making, and celebrating successes. Introducing your 4- to 6-year-old to simple household tasks sets the stage for building valuable life skills. Each task offers an opportunity for growth, whether it's sorting the laundry or feeding the family pet. Even small responsibilities provide essential opportunities for skill-building, helping them develop self-confidence and a sense of accomplishment. As they manage these tasks, your encouragement and clear instructions play a key role in keeping them motivated and engaged. The process allows you and your little one to explore strategies that best nurture their unique strengths and abilities.

In this chapter, we'll chat about real-life strategies designed to empower their development. You'll gain practical tools and techniques to support your little one in achieving greater independence and self-assurance, paving the way for a harmonious and fulfilling home environment.

Introducing Simple Household Tasks for Responsibility

Practical Tips

Encouraging responsibility in a young learner through manageable tasks is a pivotal component of fostering independence and self-confidence. As a parent, you can help your 4- to 6-year-old achieve these skills by offering appropriate, developmentally suitable tasks, providing clear guidance, and using engaging tools to maintain interest. This approach supports their development and creates a household dynamic that flows beautifully.

The first step is choosing developmentally appropriate tasks, which helps them stay engaged and avoid becoming overwhelmed. Selecting tasks suitable for their developmental stage is important for building their confidence and promoting a sense of competence. For instance, they might thrive on tasks like:

- Sorting the laundry by color
- Feeding the family pet
- Picking up their toys
- Watering houseplants
- Setting the dinner table
- Matching socks

As they master these tasks, you can gradually introduce more complex responsibilities. Take notice of their reactions and preferences, adjusting tasks as needed to ensure they remain manageable and enjoyable. Including your son or daughter in the decision-making process about which tasks they wish to take on gives them a sense of control and motivation. As they grow, consider letting them explore responsibilities such as helping with meal prep, grocery shopping, sweeping, or even making their bed.

You could even incorporate visual schedules as a great way to help with understanding and consistency. Studies show that children on the autism spectrum benefit from visual aids because they process information more clearly through images than words (Carter & Hartley, 2020). A colorful chart or planner with pictures depicting each task acts as a consistent daily reminder of responsibilities. You might design a schedule that includes illustrations of common tasks like putting away toys, feeding a pet, or setting the table. Add interactive elements such as stickers or magnets to let them track their progress independently, fostering a feeling of accomplishment. Over time, this method helps cement routines and build their organizational skills.

Involving your young learner in family chores provides an excellent opportunity to promote teamwork and a sense of belonging. When they participate in shared activities like cooking or cleaning, they gain the chance to develop valuable social skills, such as cooperation and communication.

Real Life Story: The Schultz Family

The Schultz family had always been a tight-knit crew, but when their youngest, Nole, was diagnosed with autism spectrum disorder at age 6, their lives changed in ways they hadn't anticipated. Nole, with his deep love for their family cat, Sam, struggled to stay focused during their daily routine. His parents, Jennifer and Mark, were determined to help him feel included in the family's activities, but it wasn't always easy.

Max, their oldest at 12, decided to step in with a creative solution. Knowing Nole's connection to technology and visuals, Max created a special chart on Nole's tablet, making it simple and engaging to capture his attention. The chart outlined a dinner routine: eat dinner, place your dish in the sink, then feed Sam. With pictures for each step, Max ensured the process was clear and appealing to Nole. Since Sam was part of the routine, Nole was eager to participate. The transformation was remarkable.

Each evening, Nole used the chart on his tablet to guide him. He quickly grew familiar with the process, and soon enough, the once-difficult task of staying focused during dinner became second nature. He would eat, place his dish in the sink with a smile, and immediately go over to feed Sam.

Noticing its success, the family decided to build on this. They started adding more visual tasks to Nole's tablet as his confidence grew—sorting laundry, watering plants with Dad, and even putting his toys away. After introducing each task, they evaluated Nole's progress, making adjustments as needed. At times, he rose to the challenge, and other times, he found the tasks overwhelming. This trial-and-error process helped the family refine their approach to better meet Nole's needs.

Liam, the middle brother, added encouragement to the process by cheering Nole on and offering high-fives after each completed task. It became a family affair. Tasks that once seemed daunting transformed into moments of teamwork, and the Schultz family worked together, finding new ways to integrate Nole into daily life, deepening their bond with each new milestone.

Beyond these strategies, it's important to practice patience and flexibility. Foster open-ended communication by inviting your young learner to share their preferences and any difficulties they encounter with assigned tasks. This dialogue can provide valuable insights into how to adapt your approach to better cater to their needs.

ENCOURAGING INDEPENDENT DECISION-MAKING

As you begin building confidence and critical thinking skills in your 4- to 6-year-old on the autism spectrum, it's essential to focus on empowering their decision-making abilities. By nurturing these skills early, you lay the groundwork for lifelong independence and self-assurance. Here are simple, practical strategies that can help.

Offering your child a choice between limited options simplifies decision-making and is a great starting point. Imagine a scenario where they need to choose a snack. If you open the pantry door and offer them a variety of shelves filled with options, they might become overwhelmed. Now, imagine instead that you allow them a choice between two snacks. Presenting only two options—perhaps an apple or a banana—avoids overwhelming them and makes it easier to evaluate and decide. This practice not only makes the process simpler but also allows your learner to feel a sense of control over their choices. Limiting options encourages focus and reduces anxiety, paving the way for more confident decisions.

Problem-solving through real-life scenarios is another effective approach to building critical thinking. Incorporating these scenarios into everyday learning experiences can make them engaging and relatable. For instance, if your little one encounters a toy that doesn't work, help them identify the issue and brainstorm potential solutions. You might ask questions like, "Why do you think the toy isn't working?" or "What can we do to fix it?" Encouraging your child to think critically and investigate equips them with tools to tackle challenges in the best way possible. These exercises foster problem-solving skills, boost confidence, and encourage analytical thinking, laying the groundwork for independent decision-making.

Play is a powerful tool for practicing decision-making skills safely. By engaging your 4- to 6-year-old in pretend play scenarios like running a store or hosting a picnic with toys, you create opportunities for them to make choices and express preferences within a secure environment. Through play, they learn about the relationship between cause and effect, helping them recognize the consequences of their decisions. This approach also provides a low-risk platform for experimentation, where they can test ideas without the fear of failure. Whether deciding what stuffed animal will join them at the picnic or determining how to arrange their store, these playful decisions enhance confidence, encourage self-expression, and strengthen cognitive development.

As they become more comfortable with decision-making, you can gradually increase the complexity of the choices they face. Start by introducing an additional option, then slowly layer new elements into familiar scenarios. For example, once they're adept at choosing between two snacks, you might offer three options or involve them in meal planning. This gradual escalation challenges them to weigh pros and cons and adjust to changing information, enhancing their adaptability and understanding of more complex situations. By progressively expanding their decision-making tasks, you nurture flexibility and resilience—critical traits for navigating life's challenges.

Critical thinking underpins all these activities. You can encourage your young learner to think critically about their decisions by reflecting on what worked well and areas for improvement. After resolving a toy problem, try asking them questions like, "What did we learn from fixing it? Is there something we could do differently next time?" Encouraging reflection not only reinforces their learning but also fosters a mindset focused on continuous growth. Make it a point to celebrate their successes and insights, as this strengthens positive associations with decision-making and further boosts their confidence and self-esteem.

Celebrating Small Successes to Boost Self-Esteem

Building self-esteem and motivation in your 4- to 6-year-old on the autism spectrum starts with recognizing achievements. An effective way to foster self-esteem is to focus on setting small, achievable goals. Let's say your child struggles with getting dressed independently. Begin with a task that feels manageable, like putting on their socks or pulling on a shirt. Once they manage that first sock by themselves, enthusiastically celebrate—jump up and down, clap, or give specific praise. This lets them know that every achievement counts. This process helps them realize that success isn't just about completing big projects but also involves progress through mastering smaller, incremental steps.

Story sharing is another powerful tool to foster pride. Encourage your kiddo to talk about their successes by sharing stories during family time. Start by sharing a personal achievement of your own, then gently encourage them to share one of theirs. These stories don't need to be grand accomplishments; even small wins, like learning to tie shoelaces or finishing a puzzle, deserve recognition. This practice not only boosts their confidence but also improves communication skills and strengthens family connections. Your child will begin to understand that their experiences are valuable and worth celebrating, building pride in their individuality.

Organizing family celebrations for milestones highlights the importance of recognition. Whether they've mastered a new skill or achieved a long-term goal, organizing a small family gathering can emphasize these milestones. These celebrations could be as simple as hosting a special dinner at home, baking a cake, or planning an outing to their favorite park. These events create lasting memories linked to their achievements, showing them that their hard work brings happiness not only to them but also to those they love.

As you implement these strategies, remember that consistency and sincerity in your feedback and celebrations are crucial for building their self-esteem. Avoid over-praising or offering insincere compliments, as your child may quickly recognize when praise is not genuine, potentially causing mistrust or confusion. Instead, focus on specific efforts and improvements, and acknowledge their genuine achievements honestly. Doing so builds trust and reinforces their belief in their capabilities.

Providing Practical Tools for Independence

As you begin to navigate life with your amazing child on the autism spectrum, it's essential to equip yourself with tools and strategies that promote independence and confidence. In this section, we'll touch on practical, impactful methods designed to fit seamlessly into your daily routines.

We've already emphasized the importance of visual aids, such as task charts, as powerful tools for helping your little one manage tasks more effectively. These aids work by breaking down activities into steps they can handle, allowing them to see what needs to be done and track their progress visually. When they check off completed tasks, your loved one can take ownership of their routine, which fosters a sense of accomplishment and independence. Studies have shown that visual aids enhance on-task behavior and scheduling skills (Thomas & Karuppali, 2022), thereby promoting self-reliance.

Beyond visual aids, remember the importance of consistent praise and reinforcement for building your child's confidence and responsibility. Acknowledging their efforts is crucial. This could mean congratulating them for tidying their toys or following directions without reminders. This positive reinforcement helps encourage desired behaviors and motivates them to replicate them. The key here isn't only to emphasize the outcome but also to appreciate the effort and determination your little one shows throughout the process. This encouragement builds a supportive environment where they feel valued and understood.

Putting routines in place is another powerful strategy for promoting your kid's independence and maintaining your sanity. Predictable routines provide a framework that gives structure to their day. Consistency is key—it helps reduce anxiety because they know what to expect, which is especially comforting for those who don't handle change very well. Simple routines, such as bedtime rituals or having designated meal and play times, help shape an atmosphere swirling with peace and stability. They also teach time management skills and allow your child to anticipate what comes next, giving them a sense of security and empowerment.

Another valuable tool for tracking growth is maintaining a progress journal. We've touched on this a bit, but it's worth diving in and going into more detail. This tool serves multiple purposes: It records your child's improvements over time, and acts as a motivational resource. When you document milestones—like learning new words or completing a series of tasks independently—it provides a tangible record of success that both you and your young learner can reflect on. Reviewing past achievements reinforces your loved one's accomplishments and boosts self-esteem, encouraging them to set and pursue new goals. For you, this journal offers insights into their development trajectory, highlighting areas of improvement and those that may need additional focus. Regularly updating and reviewing this journal ensures it remains relevant as your son or daughter grows and learns.

Something to consider while implementing these strategies is finding a balance between providing support and encouraging independence. While it's important to offer guidance, creating room for mistakes and learning experiences is equally important. Cheering your child on when they repeat tasks consistently instills confidence. Eventually, these activities will become second nature, reinforcing their confidence in their own abilities. By giving them opportunities to practice and succeed, you nurture their resilience and patience—qualities that will benefit them well beyond childhood.

FINAL INSIGHTS

Helping your 4- to 6-year-old on the autism spectrum gain independence and self-confidence is a process filled with many small steps that lead to much bigger things. We've gone over many strategies in this chapter, such as introducing simple household tasks to build responsibility and family involvement, like tidying up toys together or setting the table. These tasks create a strong sense of belonging and they strengthen social skills through teamwork and communication.

Remember, helping your little one develop decision-making abilities lays a foundation for future independence. Keep that patience and flexibility flowing as you adapt strategies to fit their unique needs, nurturing their growth and tightening your bond.

Next, we'll explore strategies to help your child effectively manage sensory overload in public spaces.

KEY TAKEAWAYS

- **Start with age-appropriate tasks:** Introduce simple household activities, such as feeding the family pet or tidying up toys, to foster a sense of responsibility and achievement.
- **Leverage visual aids for clarity:** Use task charts with pictures or visual schedules, such as a morning routine chart, to help your 4- to 6-year-old follow tasks and track progress effectively.
- **Gradually increase task complexity:** Begin with simple, guided choices, such as selecting between two toys, and progressively introduce more complex tasks to foster decision-making skills incrementally.
- **Celebrate every success:** Acknowledge all accomplishments, big or small, to boost self-esteem and motivation.
- **Encourage independent decision-making:** Offer structured choices, like selecting a snack or activity, to empower them with confidence in making decisions independently.

8
MANAGING SENSORY OVERLOAD IN PUBLIC PLACES

Managing sensory overload in public spaces can feel like a dynamic challenge for you as the parent of a 4- to 6-year-old child on the autism spectrum. Research shows that certain environments can become overwhelming, causing stress and discomfort that may turn fun outings into stressful experiences (Marco et al., 2011).

If you're new to this crazy little thing called parenting, balancing exposure to the outside world with your kid's comfort can feel like walking a tightrope, as public settings often heighten anxiety for both you and your little one. Managing sensory overload in these environments is about creating a sense of trust and security, helping both of you feel more at ease during outings.

It's time to jump right into this next chapter, where we'll go over strategies to support your child's sensory needs in public, empowering you to turn potentially stressful experiences into manageable and enjoyable opportunities—fostering their resilience and confidence as they engage with the world around them.

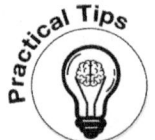 **Planning Ahead With Sensory Tool Kits**

We've discussed the importance of creating personalized sensory tool kits and how they can transform experiences for both you and your 4- to 6-year-old, especially when in public spaces. These kits are designed to equip them with tools to help manage sensory overload, turning outings into exciting experiences instead of a dreadful whirlwind of worry.

As I mentioned in Chapter 2, assembling a portable sensory tool kit with items like noise-canceling headphones, fidget toys, and weighted blankets can be highly effective in managing sensory overload. For example, noise-canceling headphones block out overwhelming sounds in noisy environments like grocery stores, giving your little one a quieter space to focus. Fidget toys, such as stress balls or pop tubes, engage their sense of touch, helping to soothe and distract from distressing stimuli. A small, weighted blanket or lap pad provides comforting deep pressure, creating a sense of security and calm, like a gentle hug.

Flexibility in selecting sensory tools allows you to customize a tool kit that fits their unique sensory needs and preferences. As your child's needs vary, so can the items, such as textured objects for tactile stimulation or gum and snacks for oral soothing. Introducing the tool kit at home in a safe and familiar environment helps build familiarity and boosts its effectiveness, making it easier for them to rely on these tools in public settings to cope effectively during outings.

Real Life Story: Sophia and Her Daughter Ella

Sophia, a first-time mom, felt her heart sink every time her daughter, Ella, had a meltdown in public. Diagnosed with autism at age 4, Ella was particularly sensitive to noisy environments, and grocery store trips often turned into overwhelming experiences. The harsh fluorescent lights, constant chatter, and hum of machinery triggered sensory overload, leaving Sophia both stressed and unsure of how to help. After one particularly difficult day, she decided something had to change. Sophia spent hours researching sensory strategies and spoke with Ella's therapist, who suggested assembling a sensory kit tailored to her needs.

Soon, Ella had her very own sensory backpack, a bright pink one she loved. Inside, Sophia included her daughter's favorite plush elephant, noise-canceling headphones to muffle loud sounds, and bubble wrap, which Ella adored for its calming pop. During their next grocery trip, everything felt different. As soon as Ella started feeling overwhelmed, she reached for her headphones, clutched her elephant, and focused on the satisfying pops of the bubble wrap. What had once been a dreaded ordeal was now manageable, and for the first time, Sophia left the store feeling hopeful rather than defeated. This simple sensory kit completely transformed their outings, giving both Sophia and Ella the tools they needed to succeed.

Preparation before visits is another key strategy. Think about the environment you're planning to visit, focusing on elements like noise level, crowd size, and available amenities. For example, visiting a museum at less crowded times reduces sensory input, making the experience more manageable. Additionally, planning shorter visits and gradually increasing the duration helps build your child's resilience and confidence in navigating different environments. Identifying potential quiet areas within a venue, such as a library room or outdoor garden, provides a retreat to ease sensory overload when it becomes too intense.

Pre-visit preparations also mean involving your child in the planning process. Empower them by discussing upcoming outings ahead of time, detailing what they might see, hear, or encounter. This can help ease anxiety about the unknown. Providing visual aids or social stories outlining the trip can further solidify expectations, helping your 4- to 6-year-old feel more prepared for the sensory inputs they may experience.

It's important to remember that each outing is a learning experience for both you and your child. Observing how they interact with their tool kit can guide future adjustments. After each outing, take a moment to discuss what items were most helpful and which ones might need tweaking. This regular feedback ensures the tool kit evolves to meet their changing needs, making each outing smoother than the last.

Identifying Safe Spaces for Breaks

Motivational Moment

Handling public spaces with your 4- to 6-year-old who may experience sensory overload can be overwhelming for any parent. Sensory overload occurs when their senses are bombarded by external stimuli, resulting in feelings of distress and being overwhelmed. These experiences may happen often and can feel especially challenging. However, recognizing and utilizing safe spaces in public environments can greatly reduce the stress of outings for both you and your little one.

Recognizing sensory-friendly locations is key if you want everything to go smoothly when out with your 4- to 6-year-old, as these places are designed to minimize sensory input and reduce the risk of overwhelming them. Venues like libraries, nature parks, and sensory-friendly cinemas tend to offer calmer environments compared to busy, crowded areas. Planning ahead by identifying these locations or choosing to visit during quieter times helps align with their sensory needs. Additionally, scheduling regular break times during outings allows your child to step away from stimulating environments and recharge, offering a sense of predictability and helping them maintain control.

To manage sensory overload, creating a sensory rescue plan can be highly beneficial. A sensory rescue plan outlines how to access designated safe spaces when out and about. This plan might involve mapping out exits, restroom locations, nearby parks or quieter areas, and identifying businesses with sensory-friendly accommodations. Having these details prepared beforehand provides peace of mind and assures both you and your child that there's a quick escape if needed. Let your brave little adventurer know that these handy sensory tools, such as noise-canceling headphones or sunglasses, will come to the rescue if they start to feel uncomfortable or stressed.

Building rapport with venue staff is another valuable approach. Friendly and informed staff members can offer quicker assistance, support, or guidance when required, making them an invaluable resource during visits to public places. Introducing yourself and your little explorer to staff upon arrival and explaining their needs fosters understanding and creates a supportive environment. Many venues train their staff to handle diverse customer needs, including those stemming from sensory sensitivities. Learning about the resources or services they offer—such as quiet rooms or special seating arrangements—could be the ultimate game changer. If your little one begins experiencing distress, having someone informed about your situation nearby can help ensure swift action to alleviate their discomfort.

To make sure you're successful in using these strategies, practicing in familiar settings doesn't make perfect necessarily, but it does make for a much smoother experience because you have a plan of action. Start by incorporating sensory-friendly elements into outings close to home. Visit parks or local community centers known for their quietness. As your child becomes accustomed to these environments, gradually introduce new places while applying the same principles, helping build their confidence and resilience over time.

Educating Your Child on Communicating Their Needs

Empowering your 4- to 6-year-old to communicate their needs during sensory overload is crucial for their well-being, especially in public spaces. As a parent navigating this journey, understanding and implementing strategies to support their ability to express themselves can make outings more enjoyable and less stressful for both of you.

Lean into visual aids like PECS from Chapter 4, cue cards, or picture communication systems. These tools are invaluable for strengthening their ability to express themselves. They provide a visual representation of feelings, needs, or requests, making it easier for them to convey what they are experiencing. A set of small cards showing different emotions or actions—like needing a break or feeling anxious—can be used by your little one to signal their needs nonverbally. When you incorporate these aids into daily routines, your child can become familiar with using them both at home and in public settings, fostering greater independence in communicating with others.

Role-playing different scenarios at home is another effective technique that helps build vocabulary and confidence for real-life situations. When you simulate potential encounters or challenges they might face in public, you can prepare them for how to handle these situations. For example, you could act out a scenario where the noise level becomes overwhelming and practice together how they might ask to move to a quieter area. This type of play-based learning not only reinforces language skills but also boosts their confidence in managing similar situations outside the home. Furthermore, it allows you to introduce new words and phrases that might be useful, ensuring your 4- to 6-year-old feels equipped and empowered to engage with the world.

Reinforcing self-advocacy skills is particularly important, as it empowers your child to view articulating when they feel overwhelmed as a strength rather than a weakness. Encourage them to acknowledge their feelings without shame and to speak up about their needs. Each time they express feeling overloaded, it becomes an opportunity to teach them that advocating for their comfort and boundaries is a positive and commendable skill. Regularly discussing and validating their experiences helps foster a positive mindset regarding self-expression. When your little one is praised for recognizing and voicing their needs, they learn to value and trust their instincts, strengthening their resilience over time.

Creating a personal mantra is another supportive strategy that can help your kiddo verbalize feelings and initiate breaks independently. A mantra is a simple phrase or sentence that they can repeat to themselves to focus and calm their mind. It could be as straightforward as "I need a moment" or "It's okay to take a break." The mantra serves as a reminder that stepping back to regroup is perfectly acceptable. Practicing this mantra at home can make it second nature for them when they feel anxious in public places. Developing this habit encourages self-regulation and gives them a sense of control over their environment and reactions.

EVALUATING AND ADJUSTING

Every outing offers valuable lessons. After you've been out, take some time to assess what worked well and what didn't. For example, ear defenders might help keep your 4- to 6-year-old calm in loud environments, while a brightly colored toy could create more distraction than comfort. Understanding these nuances allows you to make ongoing improvements and necessary adjustments. Think of it as fine-tuning an instrument: when it's well-tuned, outings become smoother and more enjoyable.

Their feedback is key to finding the right balance. Pay attention to what they communicate, whether through words or behaviors. For instance, if they often reach for a particular item in the tool kit, this suggests it's especially useful. On the other hand, if something stays untouched during multiple outings, consider removing it from the kit. Tailoring the tool kit to their experience not only strengthens its effectiveness but also empowers your child to self-soothe using their favorite and most helpful tools.

Keeping a log of your outings can be a great strategy. Write down which places triggered sensory overload and which aspects of the environment were tricky for them to handle. Tracking these details helps identify patterns over time, such as specific triggers, times of day, or situations where your little one is more likely to become stressed. This knowledge can guide you in preparing for future outings, allowing you to anticipate certain issues and adjust your approach accordingly. For example, if your log reveals that busy supermarkets are a common challenge, you might choose to visit during quieter hours or explore alternative shops with a calmer atmosphere.

Continually building on your sensory strategies requires adopting a mindset of flexibility and openness to change. What works today may not necessarily work tomorrow, as your child grows and their needs evolve. Being adaptable ensures that the support you provide remains relevant and helpful over time. You might consider sharing your observations with professionals involved in their care, such as therapists or educators, who can provide valuable insights and suggestions.

It's important to remember that you aren't alone in this journey. Joining a community of parents who share similar experiences can be an incredible experience. These groups provide a platform to exchange ideas, share tips, and seek recommendations for sensory tools and techniques. Learning from others who understand the unique challenges and triumphs of raising a kid on the autism spectrum offers both reassurance and inspiration. Joining a community of people who understand what you're going through can give you comfort in a way that sensory tools give your 4- to 6-year-old comfort when in loud or busy environments. We all need something that recenters our focus and brings us some peace now and then.

FINAL INSIGHTS

Managing public spaces with your 4- to 6-year-old can be a challenging yet rewarding experience. This chapter explored practical strategies for managing sensory overload, emphasizing the importance of creating personalized sensory tool kits and identifying safe spaces. Remember, each outing is an opportunity to learn what works best for your little one and adjust your approach as needed. It's about finding a balance between thoughtful preparation and embracing the natural unpredictability of life in public settings.

As you take these steps, you aren't just helping your child succeed in different environments; you're also fostering their confidence and independence. Celebrate each moment, knowing that every experience contributes to guiding them toward thriving confidently in a bustling world.

In the next chapter, we'll explore how to implement positive behavior strategies to encourage good behavior in your 4- to 6-year-old, supporting them in navigating their environment with greater ease and confidence.

KEY TAKEAWAYS

- **Create a personalized sensory tool kit:** Tailor a kit with items like noise-canceling headphones and fidget toys to help your 4- to 6-year-old manage sensory overload.
- **Introduce tools at home:** Familiarize your child with sensory tools in a safe, comfortable environment to build their confidence for public use.
- **Plan for outings:** Choose sensory-friendly locations and identify quiet spaces for breaks to minimize stress and avoid meltdowns.
- **Teach communication skills:** Help your child express their needs using visual aids or role-playing to boost confidence during outings.
- **Stay flexible:** Reflect on each outing, adjusting the sensory kit and strategies to meet your child's evolving needs.

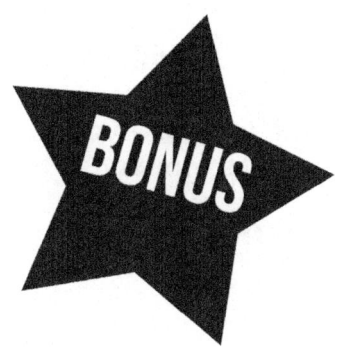

CREATE PEACEFUL MOMENTS WITH QUIET TIME MAGIC TO HELP MANAGE SENSORY OVERLOAD IN PUBLIC SPACES

Managing sensory overload can be one of the toughest challenges for your 4- to 6-year-old on the autism spectrum, especially in public spaces. That's why I've created the **Quiet Time Magic Meditation**, a free audio bonus designed to help your young learner relax and recharge.

WHAT YOU'LL GAIN

This calming meditation features:

1. **Soothing Music and Gentle Guidance**: Transition your little one into a state of relaxation with a comforting voice and calming melodies.

2. **Stress Relief Anywhere**: Use it during transitions, nap time, or even after overstimulating public outings.

3. **Reduced Anxiety**: Foster a sense of peace and security for your child.

HOW TO ACCESS QUIET TIME MAGIC

1. **Visit** https://www.parentingmasteryseries.com/autism-resource1 to download the meditation audio, or

2. Scan the QR code below:

Give your child the gift of calm today!

Warmly, Heather

9
POSITIVE REINFORCEMENT AND BEHAVIOR STRATEGIES

Implementing positive reinforcement and behavior strategies is essential for helping your 4- to 6-year-old manage and understand their environments confidently. Focusing on encouraging good behaviors tailored to your child's interests and strengths creates a more supportive and understanding atmosphere at home.

The goal of this chapter is to explore the power of positive reinforcement and how it builds self-esteem and trust. This approach emphasizes acknowledging and rewarding efforts, bolstering confidence, and making everyday interactions more meaningful for you and your young learner. By creating a nurturing space where all wins are celebrated and used as stepping stones for larger victories, you set the stage for fostering growth and a supportive environment.

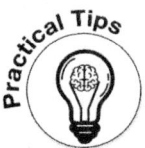

A Reward System That Will Work for Your Child

Studies have shown consistent results, indicating

that a reward system may help your 4- to 6-year-old on the autism spectrum respond positively and promote learning and social behavior (Matyjek et al., 2023). The question becomes, how can you tailor this approach to meet their unique needs?

Understanding and engaging with your little one on a personal level is crucial when developing a reward system tailored to their personal interests. Start by observing what excites them during play or activities, and consider keeping a journal to track their reactions and preferences. Once you've identified what resonates with them, create a visually engaging reward system that provides clear progress and routine, such as a sticker chart. If your 4- to 6-year-old loves animals, using animal-themed stickers can make it more appealing and reinforce positive behavior immediately. Finding something that caters to their preferences makes it a golden strategy.

Involving them in designing a personalized reward system can increase its effectiveness since they're more likely to be motivated by things they helped with. Research shows that when kids experience positive affective responses to actions, such as receiving rewards, they're encouraged to continue those behaviors over time (Van Cappellen et al., 2017). This individualized approach fosters sustained engagement and success by aligning rewards with their interests and strengths.

Setting up a tiered reward system provides a structured framework that differentiates between smaller tasks and bigger accomplishments, helping them understand varying levels of effort. For simple daily goals like feeding a pet, offer smaller rewards, such as a special sticker or bedtime story choice. For larger milestones, like mastering a new skill or completing a weekly checklist, offer bigger rewards, such as a trip to the park. Acknowledging and celebrating each success with genuine praise reinforces positive behavior, boosts their self-esteem, builds motivation, and strengthens a supportive environment.

Some practical considerations when implementing progress and routine, such as a sticker chart. If your 4- to 6-year-old loves animals, using animal-themed stickers can make it more appealing and reinforce positive behavior immediately. Finding something that caters to their preferences makes it a golden strategy.

Involving them in designing a personalized reward system can increase its effectiveness since they're more likely to be motivated by things they helped with. Research shows that when kids experience positive affective responses to actions, such as receiving rewards, they're encouraged to continue those behaviors over time (Van Cappellen et al., 2017). This individualized approach fosters sustained engagement and success by aligning rewards with their interests and strengths.

Setting up a tiered reward system provides a structured framework that differentiates between smaller tasks and bigger accomplishments, helping them understand varying levels of effort. For simple daily goals like feeding a pet, offer smaller rewards, such as a special sticker or bedtime story choice. For larger milestones, like mastering a new skill or completing a weekly checklist, offer bigger rewards, such as a trip to the park. Acknowledging and celebrating each success with genuine praise reinforces positive behavior, boosts their self-esteem, builds motivation, and strengthens a supportive environment.

Some practical considerations when implementing these strategies include starting small and gradually expanding the reward system as they becomes more comfortable with each step of the process. Focusing on one behavior at a time minimizes overwhelm and promotes success. Using clear, simple, and age-appropriate language ensures that they fully understand what's required of them. For example, try, "Can you put this book on the shelf?" rather than "Clean up this room." Keeping it simple and specific is best.

Additionally, it's important to distinguish between a reward system and bribery. While a reward system is structured around clear expectations and consistent reinforcement of desired behaviors, bribery is reactive and unplanned, which can lead to confusion and unpredictability for your learner. Instead, set clear guidelines and communicate them effectively, encouraging behaviors that are grounded in intrinsic motivation rather than relying solely on external rewards.

Integrating Positive Feedback Into Daily Schedules

Incorporating positive feedback into daily routines creates an uplifting environment for your child, encouraging growth and confidence. Establishing routine check-ins for feedback strengthens communication and interactions. These check-ins should be consistent, providing them with a reliable experience of positive reinforcement, much like a regular schedule that provides structure and predictability. By setting aside specific times to offer feedback, you create consistent opportunities to acknowledge progress, no matter how small.

Communicating through positive phrasing is another key element. This involves focusing on what they're doing well rather than emphasizing negative or undesirable behaviors. Instead of saying "Don't run," try saying "Let's try walking calmly." This approach not only reduces negativity but also demonstrates the kind of behavior you want to encourage. The language you choose shapes interactions by fostering positivity and reinforcing that they are capable and valued.

Integrating positive affirmations into everyday activities builds a habit of praise that becomes second nature. Start small by acknowledging simple achievements, whether it's completing a puzzle or showing patience while waiting. These affirmations don't need to be elaborate; even a quick; "I'm proud of how hard you tried" makes a meaningful impact on your child's self-esteem. As this practice becomes part of your daily routine, they will begin to internalize these affirmations, fostering a greater sense of worth and accomplishment.

Real Life Story: The Thompson Family

The Thompson family had been searching for ways to help their son Issaiah, diagnosed with autism at age 4, better regulate his emotions and behavior. After trying countless strategies, one thing finally clicked—daily positive affirmations.

It started simply with Dad sharing one thing he was proud of during breakfast, followed by Mom. Whether it was praising Issaiah for finishing his meal or recognizing his creativity in play, these small moments began to make a big difference. Over time, Issaiah started to expect this routine, and the day seemed to start on a brighter note.

At night, after stories, Issaiah's visual schedule featured a picture of Mom and Dad, signaling that affirmations were next. This part of the day became his favorite, as his parents each told him one reason why they loved him or were proud of him, bringing calm and always evoking a big smile.

After a year of consistently using affirmations, something wonderful happened. One evening, instead of waiting for his parents to start, Issaiah wrapped his little arms around them and whispered, "I love you." It was a breakthrough, a heartwarming moment that filled the Thompsons with joy. This practice of daily affirmations not only supported Issaiah's emotional regulation but also strengthened the family bond in meaningful ways.

The timing of feedback is essential for reinforcing desired behaviors, as offering immediate praise during or right after the action helps strengthen your child's understanding of the connection between the behavior and its positive outcome. Immediate reinforcement encourages them to associate their actions with rewards, increasing the likelihood of repeating the behavior. For example, if your child feeds the dog, praising them immediately with specific feedback, like "You did a great job feeding Rover so neatly," enhances their motivation to continue these positive actions.

Over time, this feedback loop helps develop self-motivation in them. While they may initially seek external validation through your praises, they'll gradually begin identifying ways to improve independently. This shift encourages them to take pride in their achievements and continue pursuing goals, combining the joy of receiving praise with the intrinsic satisfaction of their efforts.

It's important to acknowledge and celebrate small wins alongside larger milestones, as recognizing achievements like remaining seated during mealtime or expressing needs verbally reinforces progress. Consistently acknowledging these efforts shows your little one that growth comes from a series of small, consistent steps toward bigger goals. Positive reinforcement isn't just about compliments, but about fostering a nurturing mindset that actively supports and guides them in developing better behavioral patterns.

As you weave positive reinforcement into their daily life, keep in mind the balance and authenticity of your feedback. Your 4- to 6-year-old is remarkably intuitive and can sense insincerity. Therefore, you'll want to make sure your affirmations are both genuine and well-earned. Aim for a balance where acknowledgments are meaningful and encouraging, without becoming overwhelming or expected at every turn.

Overcoming Challenges With Encouraging Alternatives

Managing the challenges associated with autism often involves shifting focus from negative behaviors to positive alternatives. This process can benefit both you and your 4- to 6-year-old, offering more constructive ways to engage with the world around them. Understanding and identifying what triggers certain behaviors is imperative—it's often the first step in creating effective strategies to address these issues.

One practical tool you can use is a behavior diary. By

systematically recording situations that lead to specific behaviors, patterns can emerge, providing valuable insights into triggers that might not be immediately apparent. For example, you might notice that tantrums often follow transitions or occur in overwhelming environments. Identifying these moments helps pinpoint areas where targeted strategies are needed for intervention.

Once you have a clearer understanding of the triggers, it's vital to teach alternative responses. Offering choices empowers your child by giving them an active role in managing their behavior. For instance, if transitions are challenging, offer a choice between two preferred activities to help them feel in control. This approach reduces resistance and supports the development of self-regulation skills as they learn to navigate emotions in different scenarios.

Finally, don't forget to collaborate with all your son or daughter's caregivers—whether family members, educators, or therapists. This collaboration expands the range of available solutions. Sharing observations and discussing strategies with others involved in their life ensures consistency while reinforcing positive changes across different environments. A collaborative approach amplifies the impact of the strategies you implement, providing a holistic framework that nurtures growth and development.

ENGAGING WITH COMMUNITY SUPPORT AND RESOURCES

As a parent of a 4- to 6-year-old on the autism spectrum, you may often feel like you're in this alone. However, the power of community support and available resources can transform your journey by helping you face challenges collaboratively. Imagine if, instead of feeling isolated, you had a network of understanding allies eager to share experiences, offer advice, and lend a helping hand.

First, consider joining local support groups. These groups provide a safe space where you can connect with other parents who understand the unique joys and challenges you face. Sharing your story and listening to others can be cathartic and empowering. You may discover strategies that have worked for others or simply find comfort in knowing you aren't alone. Support groups often meet regularly and offer flexible scheduling to accommodate different needs. Accessing this kind of peer advice is invaluable, as it provides real-world applications from people actively navigating similar paths. For example, the Autism Society is a great resource to connect with for support and information (Autism Society, 2024).

Consulting professionals is another critical strategy. When faced with persistent behaviors that seem difficult to manage, seeking expert advice can provide customized strategies tailored to your child's unique needs. Professionals such as behavioral therapists, psychologists, or special education teachers can assess situations with fresh eyes and suggest interventions you may not have considered. By engaging a professional, you not only tap into their knowledge but also equip yourself with the confidence to implement recommended strategies. Since every child is unique, having a personalized plan can make a huge difference in promoting positive behaviors effectively.

In today's digital age, online forums and resources provide valuable opportunities for ongoing support and learning. They're particularly beneficial because they allow you to access information on your own time, making it easy to fit into your schedule. Websites dedicated to autism awareness and parenting offer articles, webinars, and virtual workshops on topics ranging from establishing daily routines to managing sensory challenges. Online communities, much like local support groups, enable you to connect with parents worldwide. They serve as excellent platforms for shared experiences and practical tips. For instance, the Family Caregiver Alliance publishes research and resources to improve the quality of life for caregivers and those they care for, including state-specific services (Family Caregiver Alliance, 2020).

Another powerful yet often underutilized resource is collaborating with other caregivers. Working together with them offers an array of opportunities to explore broader perspectives and solutions. Whether it means exchanging babysitting duties or sharing educational materials, working together can alleviate some burdens. This collaborative spirit not only helps distribute the workload but also fosters a sense of community and shared purpose. Reaching out to trusted friends or family members to form a small network of support may lead to creative problem-solving that benefits everyone involved.

It's important to recognize that understanding the world of autism goes beyond addressing challenges; it's about fostering resilience and celebrating the unique successes within your child and your family. Taking proactive steps to leverage community support and resources strengthens a sense of collaboration. Teamwork makes the dream work after all—it creates an atmosphere where both you and your child can grow and thrive.

Remember that being active in these groups and networks isn't only about receiving support, it's about giving back whenever you can. Sharing what you've learned with others enriches their journey while also strengthening yours. Every piece of advice exchanged, and every story shared, adds to the collective understanding in the autism community, building a stronger, more connected network of support.

FINAL INSIGHTS

In this chapter, we've explored the importance of creating a personalized reward system for your 4- to 6-year-old. When you focus on what truly motivates them, you unlock new ways to encourage positive behavior. We've discussed how charts or tokens can make goals tangible and relatable, providing clear progress markers that are easy for them to follow. Don't forget to tailor rewards to their interests, making the process more engaging and fun—it nurtures their growth and independence.

Incorporating positive feedback into daily routines creates an uplifting environment where your young learner feels encouraged and valued. Simple affirmations like "Great job helping clean up!" and immediate praise help connect their actions to positive outcomes, boosting self-esteem and giving them a little motivation. By working with caregivers, educators, and community resources, you can build a support system that reinforces these principles and encourages positive behaviors.

Positive reinforcement isn't just a method; it's a mindset that nurtures trust, collaboration, and emotional resilience. By weaving these principles into daily interactions, you create a foundation that supports their long-term development, both behaviorally and emotionally.

KEY TAKEAWAYS

- **Personalizing rewards to your 4- to 6-year-old's interests:** Tailor rewards to their unique preferences, like stickers of their favorite characters or extra playtime, to create a more engaging and effective system for encouraging positive behavior.
- **Use visual aids to track progress:** Implement simple tools like sticker charts or token systems to provide clear, tangible feedback. This structure makes goals easy to understand and encourages consistency.
- **Celebrating all achievements:** Recognize both small and significant accomplishments to build self-esteem and reinforce positive behaviors. Celebrate with simple praise, high-fives, or family acknowledgment.
- **Incorporate affirmations into daily routines:** Use kind and encouraging words, like "You did a great job cleaning up!" during everyday moments to create a positive atmosphere that nurtures growth.
- **Focus on structured rewards, not bribery:** Rewards work best when planned and connected to clear goals, while bribery is reactive and short-term. Structured rewards foster confidence and long-term motivation.

10
LONG-TERM GROWTH— PREPARING FOR THE FUTURE

Preparing for the future means helping your 4- to 6-year-old build the foundational skills they need to grow and thrive in their own special way. These skills enable them to approach life's challenges and navigate transitions with greater confidence while valuing their unique strengths. As a parent, you can nurture these abilities through engaging and supportive strategies that make a meaningful difference. By focusing on fostering long-term confidence and teaching practical problem-solving techniques, you'll create a foundation that supports their successful development and adaptability.

This chapter provides practical and personalized strategies to establish a solid foundation for their lifelong learning and personal growth.

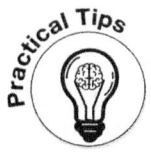

Fostering Problem-Solving Skills

Helping your 4- to 6-year-old develop essential life skills includes strengthening their problem-solving abilities, a key component when looking at the bigger picture. You play a pivotal role in nurturing this capability, which can shape how they approach challenges. Let's roll up our sleeves and uncover some practical strategies to support these skills while leveraging their unique strengths and needs.

The first step is to ignite your explorer's curiosity. Curiosity is a powerful motivator for learning and can be encouraged by engaging them in activities that align with their specific interests. Whether they love tractors, space, or art, incorporate these themes into daily activities. For example, if they are fascinated by animals, create animal-themed puzzles or interactive storytelling sessions where they can explore different scenarios and ask questions about their world. This can boost their interest in learning while laying the groundwork for developing problem-solving and critical-thinking skills. Providing opportunities for exploration makes abstract concepts easier to understand, improving comprehension and retention.

Playing games and puzzles isn't just fun for your child; studies also show these activities improve cognitive and social functioning throughout their lifetime (Atherton & Cross, 2021). These scenarios mimic real-life challenges, offering a safe space for them to experiment with solutions. Puzzles, for instance, teach patience and persistence as they work through configurations. Similarly, strategy-based board games for this age group encourage decision-making. Many educational software programs offer digital versions of these games, accommodating diverse learning styles and preferences.

Modeling transparent problem-solving processes is another effective technique. Your little one learns a great deal by observing how you approach challenges. When faced with a simple problem, verbalize your thought process aloud. Describe each step you're taking, the reasons behind it, and what you're considering. For instance, while assembling a bookshelf, you might say, "First, I'm looking at the instructions to understand the sequence." Being transparent helps them internalize the process of analyzing situations methodically, evaluating options, and choosing a course of action. This approach serves as a roadmap they can adapt to tackle their own challenges, fostering independence and confidence.

When they attempt a new puzzle or game, you'll want to praise their dedication and problem-solving attempts, regardless of the outcome. Phrases like, "I love how you tried different ways to fit that piece," or "Great job sticking with it," validate their efforts and boost confidence. Focusing on effort rather than results promotes a growth mindset, teaching them that abilities grow through practice and perseverance. Resilience becomes a natural part of their problem-solving toolkit, allowing them to tackle increasingly complex problems with confidence as they grow.

Another impactful way to build problem-solving skills is through storytelling and role-playing activities. Create scenarios that involve characters facing dilemmas, and invite your curious explorer to think of possible solutions. This approach encourages creativity and nurtures empathy as they consider different perspectives and consequences.

Additionally, digital educational games designed for skill-building are worth exploring. These games provide immediate feedback, allowing them to quickly recognize cause-and-effect relationships. This helps them adjust strategies and learn from mistakes—an essential component of developing effective problem-solving skills.

While video games sometimes attract criticism, numerous studies highlight their potential to bolster problem-solving skills by encouraging strategic thinking, creativity, and effective decision-making (Psico Smart Editorial Team, 2024). Children on the autism spectrum are often drawn to video games because they are highly visual, structured, and provide quick feedback. Playing certain video games can help your young learner develop greater flexibility in thinking, feel more comfortable with making mistakes, and understand that practice is essential for improving skills. Some examples include:

- If: A game designed to teach your child social-emotional learning skills and encourage them to reflect on their actions, understand their messages, and consider the impact of their words on others. As they advance in the game, they learn social cues and conversation techniques that help develop empathy and foster compassion.
- Minecraft: This "sandbox" game allows your young learner to take control of their environment. In creative mode, Minecraft lets them explore an unknown world, create structures, and meet animals in a safe and engaging way.

Incorporating hands-on experiences related to day-to-day life also provides meaningful opportunities for practical problem-solving practice. Engage them in activities with tangible outcomes, such as cooking a simple recipe together. Assign tasks that require planning, sequencing, and focus, like measuring ingredients or setting the table. These activities offer real-world benefits and bridge the gap between theoretical concepts and applied knowledge, helping your 4- to 6-year-old understand the relevance and value of problem-solving in everyday life.

Preparing for Life Transitions

Helping your 4- to 6-year-old prepare for larger life transitions is one of the most valuable gifts you can provide. Transitions can often feel overwhelming for them. As a parent, having a strategy in place creates smoother pathways, helping them feel more confident and secure during these changes.

In earlier chapters, we've talked about preparing your young learner for daily transitions and helping them get ready for school or social situations. It's equally important to prepare them for managing larger life transitions.

One effective method to introduce a new environment or routine is through a social story. These stories are structured narratives that describe specific situations and explain how to respond appropriately. Using social stories helps them anticipate what might happen and learn how to react in a clear and manageable way.

For instance, if they're expecting a new sibling, a personalized social story describing what to expect during the months leading up to the baby's arrival can help reduce anxiety. Doing this allows them to anticipate each step of the experience. Not only does this prepare them mentally, but it also provides a model of behavior they can emulate. Once they feel comfortable with the story, you can begin adding details about the baby coming home and what that will look like in daily life. Including familiar elements, like their name or photos, makes the story more engaging and meaningful.

Another empowering technique is practicing transition scenarios. Just like athletes rehearse before a big game, rehearsing new routines helps your child prepare for changes in a way that feels manageable and less stressful. Engage them in role-plays or practice scenarios for events like moving to a new house or going on vacation. This allows them to build confidence in a safe environment and learn at their own pace before the big event. During these practices, encourage your 4- to 6-year-old to tell you any concerns or questions they may have. This not only builds familiarity but also fosters open communication and strengthens the bond between you and them.

Visual aids, such as photos of a new home or school, can further ease transitions by helping your young learner anticipate changes.

Real Life Story: Micah and His Family

The lights were dimmed in the cozy living room as Micah snuggled between his mom and dad, his favorite blanket draped over his lap. It was story time, a cherished evening ritual, but tonight's book was special—it had been made just for him. As his mom opened the first page, bright, colorful pictures showed a mommy with a growing tummy, much like hers.

"A baby is coming to live with us, Micah," his dad said softly, "and you're going to be the best big brother." The story's pages showed pictures of the baby's room, where the baby would sleep, and the ways Micah could help—like bringing diapers, singing lullabies, and sharing gentle hugs. Micah listened intently, his eyes wide as he took in this new idea.

Over the next few months, they revisited the book nightly, each time reinforcing the excitement and answering his questions. With every reading, Micah seemed to grow more confident. He began to point to his mom's belly, asking if the baby was "in there," and he proudly showed visitors the baby's crib.

By the time his baby brother arrived, Micah was prepared. The transition, once uncertain, became a joyful family adventure. The gentle introduction of the new sibling through their special story provided Micah with a clear and comforting framework, allowing him to adjust in his own time and making the arrival of the baby a smoother experience for everyone.

Encouraging Continuous Growth

Encouraging your child's ongoing development and flexibility is a noble goal when raising a 4- to 6-year-old on the autism spectrum. As you strive to inspire continued growth, there are many personalized strategies to consider.

First, by discovering and nurturing their unique talents and interests, you pave the way for personal fulfillment and confidence. Their unique strengths—whether in music, art, technology, or nature exploration—offer meaningful opportunities for growth. By encouraging activities they already enjoy, you can uncover their natural talents. Once identified, you can encourage these talents through enriching activities, classes, or simply by providing materials at home that invite exploration.

Recognizing that learning extends beyond school boundaries is also vital in fostering a lifelong learning mindset. View education as an integral part of daily life. Encourage curiosity about the world by answering questions thoughtfully and engaging in discussions during routine activities, like grocery shopping or a walk in the park. This approach helps your child see learning as an ongoing journey rather than a destination limited to the classroom.

Establishing realistic personal growth goals is crucial in promoting perseverance. For your 4- to 6-year-old, achieving milestones can sometimes require more effort and persistence. Breaking larger goals into smaller steps makes progress seem easier to achieve. Keep celebrating their wins, as this positive reinforcement bolsters their resolve to keep pushing forward.

Another key aspect of inspiring development is promoting social connections to enhance relationships and adaptability. Social skills can be particularly challenging for your child, but they're absolutely necessary for meaningful interactions and future transitions. Encourage participation in group activities, whether it's playing a sport, joining a club, or attending community events. These settings offer opportunities to practice and refine social abilities while building friendships. You should also consider arranging playdates with friends who share similar interests, creating a safe and welcoming environment where they feel supported.

The environment in which your brave explorer learns and grows greatly impacts their development. Creating an inclusive and stimulating setting at home supports their natural curiosity and desire to learn. Allow access to a handful of resources, from books and educational toys to art supplies and digital tools that align with their interests. Regularly rotating these materials can renew their enthusiasm and encourage fresh exploration.

Communication, both verbal and nonverbal, is another area you really want to nurture. Engage in meaningful conversations and actively listen to their thoughts and feelings. Providing opportunities for expression through various mediums, including drawing, storytelling, and music, helps develop their communication skills and fosters emotional intelligence. This type of engagement builds trust and emotional connection.

Ultimately, your role as a supportive, guiding presence is central to building on your child's growth and strengthening their resilience. Balance encouragement with patience, understanding that each learner's developmental path is unique. Acknowledging setbacks as part of the process helps normalize challenges and builds confidence. Your unwavering support and always believing in them will empower them to welcome new challenges and thrive when facing adversity.

CREATING EMOTIONAL BALANCE

Continuing to promote emotional regulation in your child as they grow can be challenging and rewarding. Understanding the uncertainties that accompany this parenting journey requires thoughtful strategies and a compassionate approach. Helping them manage their emotions is crucial for their long-term growth and well-being.

First, teaching techniques for managing uncertainty transforms difficult moments into opportunities for calm and reflection. We've discussed the importance of breathing exercises, which can be introduced as a fun activity rather than a chore. Incorporating these exercises into daily routines allows them to experience their calming effects naturally over time.

Encouraging expression of emotions is another pivotal step in fostering emotional regulation. Your kid may often find it difficult to express themselves verbally, so exploring alternative outlets can be incredibly beneficial. Art, whether through drawing or painting, allows them to convey feelings when words fall short. Set aside time each week for creative sessions, offering materials like crayons, colored pencils, or paints. As they get older, journaling provides an excellent way to articulate thoughts, starting with simple prompts like "Today I feel…" or "I was happy when…"

Make it a habit to have open conversations about emotions, normalizing discussions around feelings of sadness, anger, or happiness. Constructive dialogue helps them understand that it's okay to experience a spectrum of emotions and that sharing these feelings is a healthy practice.

Validating their feelings is instrumental in normalizing their experiences of transition and growth. During moments of emotional distress, make sure they feel heard by actively listening and responding empathetically. For instance, if they seem anxious about starting a new school year, acknowledge their apprehensions with statements like, "I understand that you're feeling nervous about your first day, and that's completely normal." This affirmation reassures them that their emotions are valid and accepted. Over time, this strategy builds trust and encourages them to express their feelings without hesitation.

Incorporating mindfulness into your child's routine further solidifies these concepts. Studies show that mindfulness practices not only reduce anxiety in children on the autism spectrum but also help them become more self-aware (Loftus et al., 2023). Introduce short mindfulness exercises, such as focusing on sounds around them or feeling textures of various objects, to build self-awareness.

Similarly, implementing acknowledgment exercises, where they name and label their emotions, promotes a nonjudgmental understanding of their feelings.

FINAL INSIGHTS

In this chapter, we've explored strategies to nurture necessary skills in your 4- to 6-year-old, focusing on building long-term confidence and adaptability. These methods are designed to support their development in meaningful ways, laying a strong foundation for lifelong learning and personal growth.

We began by discussing how to build problem-solving skills by encouraging curiosity and providing structured activities like puzzles and games. These tools not only make learning enjoyable but also foster critical thinking, patience, and perseverance. Modeling problem-solving processes and reinforcing their efforts through praise helps establish a growth mindset, empowering them to tackle challenges confidently.

Next, we explored strategies for preparing your little one for life transitions. Techniques such as social stories, role-playing, and practicing new routines were highlighted as great ways to help them approach changes with reduced anxiety and greater readiness. These strategies are especially impactful when combined with visual aids and open conversations, which ensure that they feel supported and reassured throughout the process.

Fostering continuous growth was another key focus of this chapter. By nurturing your child's unique talents, encouraging curiosity beyond the classroom, and setting achievable goals, you can inspire a lifelong love of learning. Supporting social connections and providing a stimulating environment further enhance their ability to adapt and thrive.

We also emphasized the importance of emotional regulation in promoting well-being. Techniques such as breathing exercises, creative outlets, mindfulness, and open dialogue can help them navigate complex emotions with resilience. Validating their feelings and introducing calming strategies empowers your young learner to build emotional intelligence and maintain balance during life's challenges.

As a parent, your guidance and encouragement play a central role in supporting your child's long-term development. By creating an inclusive, supportive atmosphere and offering opportunities for exploration and connection, you're setting the stage for their success and adaptability. With patience and a warm, nurturing approach, you'll help them navigate the road ahead with confidence and joy.

KEY TAKEAWAYS

- **Develop problem-solving skills:** Encourage curiosity with themed puzzles, problem-solving games, or hands-on activities to build critical thinking, patience, and resilience.
- **Prepare for life transitions:** Use tools like social stories, role-playing, and visual aids to help your child approach changes with confidence and reduced anxiety.
- **Foster continuous growth:** Nurture your child's unique talents, celebrate progress, and inspire a love of learning through fun, real-world experiences.
- **Enhance emotional regulation:** Use tools like breathing exercises, creative outlets, and empathetic discussions to help your child understand and manage emotions.
- **Support long-term development:** Your encouragement and a nurturing environment ensure your little one's growth, helping them navigate each stage of life with resilience and joy.

11
SPECIAL TOPICS AND FINAL THOUGHTS

Exploring strategies for parenting your child on the autism spectrum involves understanding various modern tools and self-care techniques that can significantly support both you and your 4- to 6-year-old. With an overabundance of resources available, navigating them effectively helps you to make informed choices that cater to their unique needs. This chapter dives into how technology, self-care practices, and community networking play vital roles in crafting a nurturing environment for their development. Being mindful of these tools balances the demands of daily life while encouraging positive growth and connections.

Throughout this chapter, we'll talk about the impact of utilizing digital resources like apps designed to assist with communication, sensory management, and routine building. These tools offer creative solutions to common challenges you might face when parenting your 4- to 6-year-old, enabling smoother interactions and reducing stress for both you and them.

Utilizing Modern Apps and Online Supports

In today's rapidly advancing digital age, technology has emerged as a popular tool for parents like you. As you navigate autism parenting, it's important to explore the wealth of resources available through various digital platforms. These resources not only support your 4- to 6-year-old's development but also offer invaluable guidance and reassurance in managing daily challenges.

One important tool is communication apps, which have revolutionized how nonverbal or minimally verbal learners express their needs. Communication is a struggle for many on the autism spectrum, but apps provide customizable visuals that empower them to convey their thoughts and feelings. Using images, symbols, or recorded voice notes helps foster interaction and bridge communication gaps. For instance, apps such as Socky by Ola Mundo facilitate remote communication through illustrations, offering an effective way for minimally verbal children to interact with family members (Ash, 2024).

Sensory-friendly apps are another digital resource that can greatly benefit neurodivergent learners. These apps are designed to create calming environments by using visual schedules and structured activities that reduce anxiety. Visual schedules help young learners anticipate transitions and minimize stress caused by unexpected changes. By providing clear expectations, these apps contribute to a more predictable routine that enhances their sense of security. Apps that integrate relaxation techniques, like guided meditations or soothing sounds, are particularly effective in managing sensory overload (Rudy, 2024).

Social skills training apps are key for teaching 4- to 6-year-olds how to handle social interactions. These apps simulate real-life scenarios where they can practice responding to different social cues and situations through role-playing exercises. Engaging in these interactive sessions allows your learner to develop skills that are pivotal for building relationships and communicating effectively in various settings. Apps like ConversationBuilder are designed to improve conversation skills through themed scripts, making them effective tools for practicing socialization (Rudy, 2024).

In addition to apps directly helping your little one, parent support forums offer a layer of emotional and practical support for caregivers. These online communities connect families navigating similar journeys, providing emotional reassurance, advice on behaviors, and recommendations for local resources. A great place to start is with the National Autism Parents Forum, which is easily accessible and connects you to reputable resources in your area (Autism Parents Forum, 2024).

Embracing technology's potential allows you to better manage the unique needs of your learner while reducing stress for your family.

Prioritizing Parent Self-Care

While parenting a 4- to 6-year-old on the autism spectrum, self-care isn't just beneficial; it's fundamental for the well-being of your entire family. When you prioritize caring for yourself, you not only replenish your energy but also create a positive environment for your little one.

Mindfulness practices stand out as an effective way to manage stress. They encourage you to be present in the moment, which can help you respond rather than react to challenging situations. You can practice the same deep breathing exercises you may have already taught your 4- to 6-year-old to boost clarity and create a calm refuge during those high-stress moments. Practicing mindfulness is about finding a few minutes each day to remind yourself to breathe a little. This might include trying a technique like finger breathing, where you trace your fingers while inhaling and exhaling. These small practices can make all the difference, reducing stress and paving the way for clearer communication and decision-making.

Time management techniques are another way for parents managing the complexities of raising a young learner. Effective time management helps you carve out personal time for yourself within the demands of caring for them. By planning your day carefully, you prevent burnout and maintain harmony in your household. Consider scheduling pockets of time in your day dedicated solely to activities that refresh you, whether it's a quiet walk, reading, or a hobby you enjoy. An organized schedule allows for greater flexibility when unexpected challenges arise, saving you from feeling overwhelmed.

Professional support is invaluable when developing tailored coping strategies. Access to professionals who understand your situation offers new perspectives on handling parenting challenges unique to autism. Therapists, counselors, and special educators can offer advice customized to your family's needs, equipping you with tools that foster resilience and patience. Professional guidance can illuminate paths you might not have previously considered, ensuring you feel confident and supported in your parenting journey.

Engaging with your community holds so much value. It combats feelings of isolation by connecting you with others who know what you're going through. Joining local parent groups provides a sense of belonging and opens up opportunities for exchanging insights and advice. These groups provide emotional support and enrich your parenting strategies.

Being actively involved in community events opens your eyes to diverse perspectives and solutions. Libraries, community centers, and online forums frequently host meetings and workshops designed for parents like you. These gatherings offer more than just emotional support; they're rich with practical insights into advocacy, education, and handling systems like healthcare and schooling. When you participate in these spaces, you not only build a network but also gather invaluable resources to help your child grow.

Real Life Story: The Williams Family

The Williams family had been so focused on their autistic son's needs that they hadn't realized how much they were neglecting their own well-being. Their 4-year-old son, Ethan, often required constant attention, and the stress of handling his sensory sensitivities and meltdowns had left both parents feeling physically and emotionally drained.

After a particularly challenging week, they sat down together and admitted they were feeling completely exhausted. It was then that Ethan's therapist gently suggested they prioritize self-care, not just for themselves, but as a way to better support Ethan's needs.

Jack, Ethan's father, began practicing mindfulness, finding that taking just 10 minutes each morning for deep breathing exercises helped him stay calm during Ethan's toughest moments. Meanwhile, Emma, his mother, found comfort in participating in parenting forums and speaking to a therapist, where she could connect with others facing similar challenges. Journaling became her personal outlet, helping her process emotions and reflect on their parenting journey.

Together, they realized that by caring for themselves, they were able to approach their roles as parents with more patience, strength, and compassion, which ultimately fostered a calmer and more supportive environment for Ethan.

NETWORKING AND FORMING SUPPORTIVE COMMUNITIES

Social media communities have become indispensable tools for modern connection and support. Platforms like Facebook, Instagram, or specialized forums offer broad access to like-minded individuals, providing quick feedback on parenting challenges. Becoming a part of these online communities lets you connect with a global network of families who can empathize with your situation. Whether you're seeking advice on behaviors, educational resources, or handling transitions, social media provides a wealth of knowledge.

These interactions introduce you to varied experiences and innovative strategies you might not encounter locally. That said, always ensure the credibility of any advice obtained online and consult professionals for critical decisions regarding your child.

Parent workshops and conferences are invaluable opportunities to gain crucial insights for school preparedness and beyond. These events often feature experts in autism, including educators, therapists, and researchers, who share cutting-edge techniques and findings. Attendees gain firsthand knowledge on topics such as understanding educational rights and developing individualized education programs (IEPs) tailored to your child's unique strengths and needs.

Workshops often include interactive sessions where parents can role-play scenarios, ask questions, and take part in group discussions. This hands-on approach ensures that shared strategies are practical and applicable to everyday parenting. Conferences also serve as networking hubs, enabling you to build relationships with professionals who may later become essential allies in supporting your young learner's development.

We've discussed the importance of sharing information between home and school to help educators understand your little one's unique preferences and triggers. Regular communication with teachers helps them tailor teaching methods and daily routines, fostering a supportive learning environment. Being actively involved in IEP meetings and other school-related planning ensures that you advocate effectively for your child's needs.

Integrating Broader Technology for Effective Parenting

The digital realm offers expanded access to support, connecting you with resources and communities you might not have discovered otherwise. Online platforms allow you to share experiences and gain advice from parents worldwide who relate to your journey. These communities offer a wealth of diverse perspectives and creative solutions that can enrich your family's experience.

For instance, parents in different countries may be using innovative approaches or accessing autism research unavailable in your region. Connecting with these parents through global forums not only broadens your knowledge but also fosters a supportive network of individuals who genuinely empathize with your challenges.

Continuous engagement with technological advancements keeps you informed about best practices in autism care. For example, video modeling has emerged as a valuable tool for skill-building. Your child can watch videos demonstrating social interactions or desired behaviors, reinforcing learning in a visually engaging format. Over time, this technique helps improve communication, adaptive behaviors, and social skills in practical, everyday scenarios.

It's important to find the right balance when integrating assistive technology. While technology offers tremendous potential, it should complement—not replace—personal interaction and professional guidance. Ensuring responsible use, such as managing screen time and integrating tech tools into broader therapeutic frameworks, is vital. Remember, your child's needs are unique, and their technological requirements will vary. Tailoring tech usage to fit their specific needs optimizes its impact on both their development and your family's life.

Consider a range of solutions, from low-tech options like picture boards for foundational communication to mid-tech tools such as speech therapy apps for language development, and high-tech possibilities like virtual reality therapy brighten those social skills. The spectrum of available technologies ensures personalized interventions that align with your kiddo's learning style.

When thoughtfully embraced, technology shifts from novelty to necessity—a big component in creating a nurturing environment for your little one's growth and well-being.

FINAL INSIGHTS

In this final chapter, I've shared how modern technology, self-care practices, and community connections serve as invaluable allies in your journey of parenting your 4- to 6-year-old child on the autism spectrum. These tools and strategies work together to ease daily routines, enhance development, and strengthen emotional well-being for both you and your little one.

We began by exploring the role of modern apps and digital tools, which offer practical support in areas like communication, sensory management, and social skills training. Apps tailored to your child's needs provide interactive ways to navigate common challenges and push for independence and confidence. Equally important are online communities and forums where you can connect with other parents, exchange ideas, and find reassurance in shared experiences.

Next, we highlighted the importance of prioritizing self-care as a parent. Caring for yourself is essential in maintaining the energy and resilience required for parenting. Techniques such as mindfulness, time management, and seeking professional support create a foundation for balance and harmony in your household. By taking care of yourself, you ensure your little adventurer thrives in a nurturing and stable environment.

We also discussed the power of community—both online and offline—in providing emotional support, practical advice, and advocacy tools. From parent workshops to conferences, these resources enrich your knowledge and connect you with experts and peers who can guide and support you on this journey.

Finally, we explored the transformative role of technology in autism parenting. From video modeling and assistive communication devices to virtual reality and low-tech solutions, integrating technology in intentional and personalized ways helps your child develop vital skills while making daily life more manageable. Balancing these tools with direct interaction and professional guidance ensures their unique needs are met holistically.

KEY TAKEAWAYS

- **Leverage digital tools:** Explore apps like video modeling, communication apps, or sensory regulation devices to help your 4- to 6-year-old navigate daily life with greater ease.
- **Prioritize parent self-care:** Use mindfulness, professional support, and time management to manage stress and create a stable, nurturing environment.
- **Build a support network:** Connect with forums, local groups, or events to gain insights, build support, and feel less alone.
- **Use technology as a parenting aid:** Balance technology with personal interaction by integrating tools like assistive communication devices and low-tech solutions into your child's routine.
- **Tailor interventions to your child:** Personalize tools and strategies to meet your child's unique sensory and developmental needs, promoting their growth and well-being.

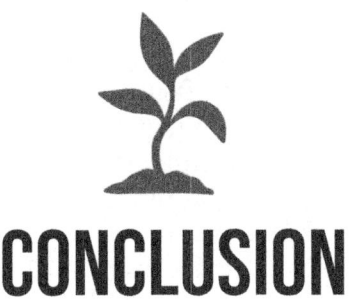

CONCLUSION

As you turn the last pages of this guide, take a moment to reflect on everything you've learned about yourself, your 4- to 6-year-old, and your uniquely beautiful ongoing adventure with autism. Every step you've taken is a testament to your unwavering commitment and love as a parent. Remember that no two families experience autism in exactly the same way; your story is your own, filled with triumphs, challenges, and endless learning opportunities.

Think back to moments where a breakthrough happened—perhaps when your young learner managed to communicate their needs effectively for the first time or demonstrated emotional resilience in unfamiliar situations. These milestones aren't just wins for them but also a validation of your efforts and dedication. Cherish these precious moments and let them remind you of the immense progress possible through patience and persistence.

The strategies and techniques outlined in this book aren't one-time solutions, they're ongoing tools for continuous development. Embrace consistency in applying what you've learned. Regularly revisit emotional regulation methods and sensory routines, and make communication a central component of your parenting approach. You might consider doing something like setting aside dedicated family time to discuss and celebrate your 4- to 6-year-old's social and emotional achievements weekly. Such repeated reinforcement will promote an environment where growth is a shared family journey.

Communication isn't only fundamental between you and your child but also crucial with caregivers, educators, and professionals involved in their life. Create a supportive environment at home where they feel comfortable expressing thoughts and emotions freely. Encourage open dialogue, showing them that their feelings matter. Imagine those cherished moments when they volunteer how happy they feel doing a particular activity with you. Those conversations offer incredible insight into their world and create deeper connections.

Building a network of support can provide invaluable resources and encouragement. Don't hesitate to reach out to local autism groups, online forums, or community workshops. Hearing other parents' stories can bring comfort and inspire you to incorporate new strategies. When you share experiences, you'll realize you're part of a larger community that is walking down a similar path, offering strength in numbers.

Keep an open mind about adapting strategies as your child grows. Their needs will evolve, and being flexible will prepare you for addressing new challenges. Consider your approach as dynamic; initially focusing on sensory routines, and then later integrating more complex social strategies as they mature. Each phase brings fresh opportunities for connection and growth, allowing both you and your young learner to adapt together.

Throughout this book, we've explored ways to balance fostering your 4- to 6-year-old's skills while maintaining your own well-being. Don't overlook your personal health and happiness amid caregiving responsibilities. Practice self-

CONCLUSION

compassion regularly—it's essential for sustaining your ability to meet their needs effectively. Try mindfulness exercises to center yourself, and don't hesitate to seek help when feeling like you have too much on your plate.

In managing the path of parenting a 4- to 6-year-old on the autism spectrum, focus on understanding both their strengths and needs. Equipped with insights into how autism manifests differently for every child, and supported by actionable advice throughout these pages, you can move forward with a realistic sense of empowerment rather than anxiety. By debunking myths and adjusting expectations based on accurate knowledge, you're better prepared to support your loved one's overall well-being and development.

Getting involved in activities that build communication and social interaction remains key. For example, using play, pictures, or simple phrases can greatly influence how your young learner interacts with the world around them. Advocate for practices within educational settings that align with these approaches to ensure continuity and reinforce progress made at home.

If progress seems stalled or inconsistent, resist discouragement. Parenting is full of ups and downs, especially with autism in the picture. Instead, view these moments as opportunities to reassess and fine-tune your techniques. Ask for professional guidance if necessary and trust in the adaptability and resilience of both you and your child.

Finally, recognize the significance of developing independence, self-confidence, and positive behaviors in your 4- to 6-year-old. Establish routines and transition strategies that make real-world interactions manageable and rewarding for them. Prepare them gradually for transitions, such as entering school, by introducing elements of change in a supportive manner. This gradual approach helps them face future challenges with greater confidence.

Parenting is ongoing and filled with continuous discovery.

Give yourself a pat on the back for your accomplishments so far and look toward future possibilities with hope and determination. Keep nurturing your relationship, grounded in love and understanding, and trust that your unique path will lead you to unexpected and extraordinary places.

If you've found this guide to be helpful in parenting your 4- to 6-year-old on the autism spectrum, I kindly encourage you to leave a review. Your feedback not only helps others discover this resource but also creates a ripple effect of shared learning and connection within the autism parenting community.

Thank you for welcoming this guide into your life. May it serve as a trusted companion, inspiring confidence, joy, and a profound sense of connection as you walk hand-in-hand with your young learner toward a strong and bright future.

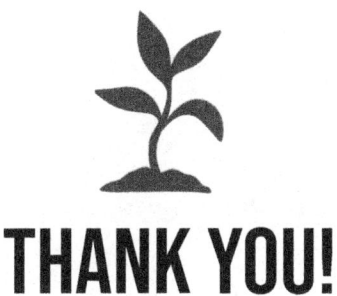

THANK YOU!

Thank you for reading *The Ultimate Guide to Parenting Your Child With Autism (Ages 4 to 6)*. Your dedication to empowering their unique journey is truly inspiring. Every step you've taken reflects your unwavering commitment to their growth, well-being, and success.

Visit to access: https://www.parentingmasteryseries.com/autism

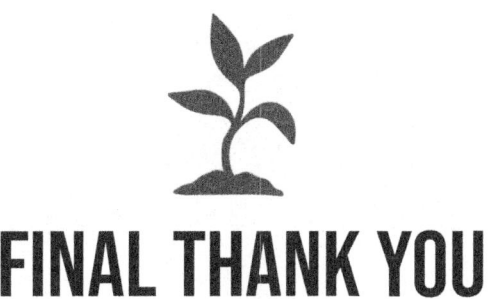

FINAL THANK YOU

Thank you again for allowing this guide to accompany you on your parenting journey. Together let's walk hand-in-hand toward a strong and bright future for your child.

Warm regards,
Heather Kingsley. Author,
Autism Parenting Mastery Series

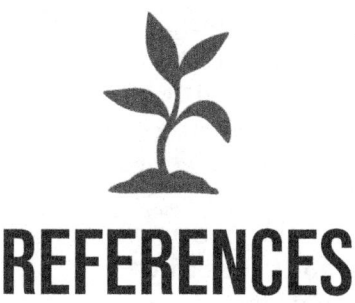

REFERENCES

ABA strategies and techniques. (2024, May 17). Special Learning.
Adina ABA Staff. (2024, July 26). What are autism behavior problems? Adina ABA.
Ash. (2024). 23 top apps for autism. Autism 360™.
Atherton, G., & Cross, L. (2021). The use of analog and digital games for autism interventions. Frontiers in Psychology, 12.
Autism Parents Forum. (2024). Autism Parents Forum.
Autism society. (2022). Autism Society.
Autism spectrum disorder: Communication problems in children. (2020, April 13)
. NIDCD. https:// autism-spectrum-disorder-communication-problems-children
Bilodeau, E. (2024, October 9). Tips for children with sensory overload in public spaces—skill point therapy. Skill Point Therapy.
Building effective communication between patients and caregivers. (n.d.). Cedar Hill Care.
Carter, C. K., & Hartley, C. (2020). Are children with autism more likely to retain object names when

learning from colour photographs or black-and-white cartoons? Journal of Autism and Developmental Disorders.

Chowdhury, M. (2019, August 13). Emotional regulation: 6 key skills to regulate emotions. Positive Psychology.

Cleveland Clinic. (2022, March 18). What is sensory play? The benefits for your child and sensory play ideas. Cleveland Clinic Health Essentials.

Customized support: Tailoring autism behavior interventions for success. (2024, February 18). ABA Building Blocks.

Daniolou, S., Pandis, N., & Znoj, H. (2022). The efficacy of early interventions for children with autism spectrum disorders: A systematic review and meta-analysis. Journal of Clinical Medicine, 11(17), 5100. https://doi.org/10.3390/jcm11175100

Dodman, E., Pena, M., & Shafai, F. (2024). Sensory processing differences toolkit. Default.

Family caregiver alliance. (2020). Caregiver.

Fernández Cerero, José, Rueda, M., & Meneses, L. (2024). The impact of parental involvement on the educational development of students with autism spectrum disorder. Children, 11(9), 1062.

Franz, L., Goodwin, C. D., Rieder, A., Matheis, M., & Damiano, D. L. (2022). Early intervention for very young children with or at high likelihood for autism spectrum disorder: An overview of reviews. Developmental Medicine & Child Neurology, 64(9), 1063–1076.

Gill, A. (2024, April 23). 12 best communication activities for kids of all ages. SplashLearn Blog.

Gonyon, A. (2023, February 1). Sensory seeking vs avoiding. Lighthouse Autism Center.

Heffron, C. (2017, September 12). 10 calming techniques and transition strategies for kids. The Inspired Treehouse.

How to support emotional regulation for kids. (2024, April 25). Sedonasky.

How toys can help develop your child's emotional intelligence. (2024, February 12). Melissa & Doug.

Ibañez, L. V., Kobak, K., Swanson, A., Wallace, L., Warren,

REFERENCES

Z., & Stone, W. L. (2018). Enhancing interactions during daily routines: A randomized controlled trial of a web-based tutorial for parents of young children with ASD. Autism Research, 11(4), 667–678.

Ilyka, D., Johnson, M. H., & Lloyd-Fox, S. L. (2021). Infant social interactions and brain development: A systematic review. Neuroscience & Biobehavioral Reviews, 130, 448–469.

Khatab, S., Fadi, H., Othman, A., & Al-Thani, D. (2024). Collaborative play for autistic children: A systematic literature review. Entertainment Computing, 50(100653), 100653–100653. https://doi.org/10.1016/j.entcom.2024.100653

Kulman, R. (2023, October 4). Making popular video games good for kids affected by autism. Autism Parenting Magazine.

Kumm, A. J., Viljoen, M., & de Vries, P. J. (2021). The digital divide in technologies for autism: Feasibility considerations for low- and middle-income countries. Journal of Autism and Developmental Disorders, 52, 2300–2313.

Loftus, T., Mathersul, D. C., Ooi, M., & Yau, S. H. (2023). The efficacy of mindfulness-based therapy for anxiety, social skills, and aggressive behaviors in children and young people with Autism Spectrum Disorder: A systematic review. Frontiers in Psychiatry, 14.

Magro, K. (2016, August 27). I want to see more autism acceptance in schools to help put an end to bullying. Kerry Magro. https://kerrymagro.com/that-moment-when-a-child-is-cruel-to-someone-with-autism/

Maksimović, S., Marisavljević, M., Stanojević, N., Ćirović, M., Punišić, S., Adamović, T., Đorđević, J., Krgović, I., & Subotić, M. (2023). Importance of early intervention in reducing autistic symptoms and speech-language deficits in children with autism spectrum disorder. Children, 10(1), 122.

Marco, E. J., Hinkley, L. B., Hill, S. S., & Nagarajan, S. S. (2011). Sensory processing in autism: A review of

neurophysiologic findings. Pediatric Research, 69(5 Part 2), 48–54.
https://doi.org/10.1203/pdr.0b013e3182130c54

Marsh, A., Spagnol, V., Grove, R., & Eapen, V. (2017). Transition to school for children with autism spectrum disorder: A systematic review. World Journal of Psychiatry, 7(3), 184–196.

Matyjek, M., Bayer, M., & Dziobek, I. (2023). Reward responsiveness in autism and autistic traits—Evidence from neuronal, autonomic, and behavioural levels. NeuroImage: Clinical, 38, 103442.

Mazefsky, C. A., Herrington, J., Siegel, M., Scarpa, A., Maddox, B. B., Scahill, L., & White, S. W. (2013). The role of emotion regulation in autism spectrum disorder. Journal of the American Academy of Child & Adolescent Psychiatry, 52(7), 679–688. https://doi.org/10.1016/j.jaac.2013.05.006

Morin, A. (n.d.). Sensory seeking vs. sensory avoiding in children. Understood.

NAMI: National alliance on mental illness. (2022). NAMI: National Alliance on Mental Illness.

National Autistic Society. (2020, August 21). Visual supports. National Autistic Society.

National Institutes of Health. (2017, January 31). Early intervention for autism.

Neff, M. (n.d.). Build a sensory self-soothing kit. Insights of a Neurodivergent Clinician.

Pfeiffer, B. A., Koenig, K., Kinnealey, M., Sheppard, M., & Henderson, L. (2011). Effectiveness of sensory integration interventions in children with autism spectrum disorders: a pilot study. The American Journal of Occupational Therapy: Official Publication of the American Occupational Therapy Association, 65(1), 76–85. https://doi.org/10.5014/ajot.2011.09205

The picture exchange communication system (PECS). (2024). National Autism Resources.

Psico Smart Editorial Team. (2024, August 28). The effect of video games on cognitive skills development and assessment. Psico-Smart.

REFERENCES

https://psico-smart.com/en/blogs/blog-the-effect-of-video-games-on-cognitive-skills-development-and-assessment-162534

Rudy, L. J. (2024, July 11). 11 apps for people with autism and their caregivers. Verywell Health.

7 tips to help your child through separation anxiety at school. (n.d.). Greenvaleschool.org.

Soto-Icaza, P., Aboitiz, F., & Billeke, P. (2015). Development of social skills in children: neural and behavioral evidence for the elaboration of cognitive models. Frontiers in Neuroscience, 9(333).

Thomas, N., & Karuppali, S. (2022). The efficacy of visual activity schedule intervention in reducing problem behaviors in children with attention-deficit/hyperactivity disorder between the age of 5 and 12 years: A systematic review. Journal of the Korean Academy of Child and Adolescent Psychiatry, 33(1), 2–15. https://doi.org/10.5765/jkacap.210021

Tracking progress in autism therapy. (2024, July 27). Goldstar Rehab.

Using visual supports in autism. (2024, June 28). Apexaba.

Van Cappellen, P., Rice, E. L., Catalino, L. I., & Fredrickson, B. L. (2017). Positive affective processes underlie positive health behaviour change. Psychology & Health, 33(1), 77–97.

Printed in Dunstable, United Kingdom